# The nurse

# in Neurology

# THE COMPLETE GUIDE

*ALEXANDRE CAREWELL*

2

# Table of Contents

*« Every action, every movement, even the most elementary thought, is a prodigy in itself. It is the result of the extraordinary synchronisation of billions of neurons. »*

# Chapter 1:
# INTRODUCTION TO NEUROLOGY

## A brief history of neurology

Neurology, that fascinating medical discipline concerned with the study of the nervous system, has travelled a long and complex road through the ages to arrive at today's understanding of the mysteries of the brain and nerves. Let's immerse ourselves in this story, which is much more than a simple chronology of events, as it reflects the evolution of our understanding of ourselves.

In ancient times, the Egyptians, Greeks and Romans laid the foundations of what was to become neurology. The Egyptians, for example, already had advanced anatomical knowledge, as witnessed by the famous Edwin Smith papyrus, which mentions observations of traumatic brain injuries. However, it was Hippocrates, the father of medicine, who asserted in the 5th century BC that it was the brain, and not the heart, that was the seat of our emotions and thoughts. A revolutionary idea at the time!

Over the centuries, with the advent of the Renaissance, the study of the nervous system was gradually refined thanks to pioneers such as Leonardo da Vinci, who produced detailed sketches of the human brain. However, it was in the 17th century, with the work of Thomas Willis, often referred to as the "father of neurology", that the discipline really took off. Willis not only identified and named several brain structures, but also laid the foundations for a clinical approach to neurological examination.

The modern era of neurology began in earnest in the 19th century, a period of scientific effervescence when technology and curiosity converged to unlock the secrets of the brain. Iconic figures such as Jean-Martin Charcot and Sir William Gowers not only defined many of the neurological diseases we recognise today, but also laid the foundations for the clinical and diagnostic principles of modern neurology.

The twentieth century saw a revolution in the understanding and treatment of neurological diseases. The discovery of electroencephalography, the introduction of magnetic resonance imaging (MRI) and advances in genetics have all opened up unprecedented insights into the functioning and dysfunction of the nervous system.

Today, neurology is at a crossroads between tradition and innovation. It draws on its rich past, while looking resolutely to the future, with the promise of gene therapies, neuroprostheses and other advances that seem straight out of a science fiction novel.

So, far from being a static discipline, neurology is a living, constantly evolving field, reflecting humanity's relentless quest to understand the most mysterious and complex organ in our body: the brain.

## The main neurological diseases

Although neurology is a specialised branch of medicine, it covers an impressive spectrum of diseases affecting the nervous system. These astonishingly diverse conditions are as varied in their symptoms as they are in their origins. Understanding them is, in a sense, trying to decipher the enigmas of our brain and our entire nervous system.

**Cerebrovascular accident (CVA)** is undoubtedly one of the best-known disorders. It occurs when blood flow to or within the brain is interrupted, depriving neurons of oxygen and causing damage, sometimes irreversible. The main types of stroke are ischaemic stroke, caused by a blood clot blocking a blood vessel, and haemorrhagic stroke, caused by the rupture of a blood vessel.

**Alzheimer's disease, a** degenerative form of dementia, takes a heavy toll on memory, reasoning and behaviour. It creeps in slowly, gradually eroding the minds and personalities of sufferers. It is characterised by the abnormal accumulation of proteins in the brain, forming plaques and tangles.

**Multiple sclerosis is an** autoimmune disease in which the immune system attacks the myelin sheath that surrounds neurons, disrupting the transmission of electrical signals. It often progresses in relapses, with periods of remission.

**Parkinson's disease**, another neurodegenerative disorder, affects movement. It is caused by the progressive death of dopamine-producing neurons in the brain. Tremors, rigidity and bradykinesia are the main signs.

**Epilepsy** refers to a series of disorders characterised by recurrent seizures. These seizures are caused by sudden electrical overactivity in the brain. They can manifest themselves in a variety of ways, ranging from momentary absence to violent convulsions.

**Migraine,** more than just a headache, is a chronic neurological disorder. It manifests itself as attacks of intense headache, often accompanied by nausea, vomiting and increased sensitivity to light or noise.

Other conditions, such as **peripheral neuropathy**, **myasthenia gravis** and **brain tumours**, illustrate the diversity of diseases that neurology must cover.

These diseases, each in its own way, are a reminder of just how robust and fragile our nervous system can be at the same time. They also underline the importance of ongoing research to better understand them and, hopefully, one day overcome them once and for all.

# The importance of the neurology nurse

The neurology nurse is a key player, often on the front line when it comes to the unique challenges posed by disorders of the nervous system. Their role is not simply a series of technical tasks, but is part of a human and therapeutic dimension that is essential to the care of patients suffering from neurological diseases.

**1. Clinical monitoring:** Neurological patients may present with subtle or sudden clinical symptoms and signs, such as changes in motor function, speech, cognition or the senses. Thanks to their training and experience, nurses are able to detect these changes, which are sometimes imperceptible to the uninitiated, and alert the medical team in good time.

**2. Treatment administration: Whether** administering anticonvulsant drugs, dopaminergic treatments or intrathecal injections, the nurse plays a crucial role. They not only ensure that the treatment is administered correctly, but also monitor the side effects and effectiveness of the treatment.

**3. Education and support:** Understanding neurological disease, its implications and treatment can be a daunting task for patients and their families. The nurse acts as a bridge, offering clear explanations, answering questions and reassuring the patient.

**4. Rehabilitation:** In conditions such as post-stroke or post-brain surgery, the nurse works closely with physiotherapists, speech therapists and other rehabilitation professionals to ensure that the patient recovers to the best of their ability.

**5. Pain management:** Many neurological conditions can be painful, from neuropathic pain to chronic headaches. Nurses play an essential role in assessing this pain and administering appropriate analgesic treatments.

**6. Emotional support:** Confronting a neurological disease can be destabilising and anxiety-provoking. Nurses offer emotional support, listening to patients, reassuring them and helping them through this difficult period.

**7. Interdisciplinary collaboration:** In neurology, patient care is often the result of collaboration between various specialists. The nurse facilitates this collaboration, ensuring fluid and effective communication between the various parties involved.

The neurology nurse, through his or her expertise, compassion and dedication, is much more than a medical auxiliary. They are the guardians of patients' well-being, the architects of their recovery, and daily witnesses to human strength and resilience in the face of neurological adversity. Their value is inestimable, making them an essential pillar of neurological care.

# Chapter 2:
# THE ENVIRONMENT
# OF THE NEUROLOGY DEPARTMENT

## Organisation and structure
## a neurology department

The Neurology Department is a complex entity that requires rigorous coordination and structuring to meet the specific needs of patients with neurological disorders. Each element of this organisation works together to provide holistic, multidimensional care.

1. Reception and assessment areas:
   - **Neurological emergency unit:** Dedicated to treating emergencies such as strokes or acute epileptic seizures.
   - **Outpatient consultations:** For patients requiring regular follow-up without hospitalisation.
2. Specialist care units:
   - **Stroke unit:** Specifically for stroke patients, with dedicated equipment and team.
   - **General neurology unit:** For a wide range of neurological diseases.
   - **Movement disorders unit:** Focuses on conditions such as Parkinson's disease.
   - **Neuroimmunology Unit:** For diseases such as multiple sclerosis.
3. Diagnostic platforms:
   - **Neurophysiology laboratory:** where EEG, EMG and other diagnostic tests are carried out.
   - **Medical imaging:** Offering MRIs, scans and sometimes PET scans, essential for diagnosing many neurological pathologies.

4. Re-education and rehabilitation services:
Focused on the functional recovery and rehabilitation of patients, these services include physiotherapy, speech therapy, physiotherapy and many others.

5. Spaces for support and well-being:
- **Rest rooms:** For patients and their families.
- **Counselling areas:** For psychological support and guidance.

6. The medical team:
- **Neurologists:** The department's pilots, specialists in neurological diseases.
- **Neurology nurses:** Dedicated to the day-to-day care and monitoring of patients.
- **Laboratory technicians:** For specialist diagnostics.
- **Caregivers:** Providing basic care and support.
- Occupational therapists, physiotherapists and other rehabilitation specialists: Essential for patients' functional recovery.
- **Neuropsychologists:** Focused on the cognitive and emotional aspects of neurological disorders.
- **Social workers:** Help patients and their families navigate the non-medical challenges associated with the disease.

7. Research and development:
In university centres and certain hospitals, research units are dedicated to the study of neurological diseases, looking for new treatments and therapeutic approaches.

The structure of a neurology department is like a well-tuned orchestra: each component, each individual, has its specific role, but all work together in harmony for the well-being and recovery of patients. Their common goal is to provide comprehensive care, from initial diagnosis through to rehabilitation, guaranteeing the best possible outcome for every patient.

# The medical and paramedical team : roles and interactions

In a neurology department, the medical and paramedical team is a heterogeneous group of professionals who, despite having different skills, work together to provide optimum patient care. Understanding the role of each member and how they interact is essential to understanding the overall dynamics of the department.

1. Neurologists:
   - **Role:** These are specialists in neurological disorders. They assess, diagnose, treat and monitor patients.
   - **Interactions:** They work closely with the nurses to monitor the patient's progress, with the laboratory technicians to interpret test results, and with the rehabilitation team to draw up appropriate care plans.
2. Neurology nurses:
   - **Role:** They are responsible for day-to-day care, clinical monitoring, administering treatments and often patient education.
   - **Interactions:** The nurses are in constant communication with the neurologists about the patients' condition. They also work in synergy with the Caregivers and collaborate with the rehabilitation specialists.
3. Laboratory technicians:
   - **Role:** They carry out diagnostic tests such as EEG and EMG.
   - **Interaction:** They provide the results to the neurologists for interpretation and work with the nurses to carry out the tests.
4. Caregivers:
   - **Role:** They provide basic care, help with patient mobility, hygiene and nutrition.

- **Interaction:** They work under the supervision of nurses and are in frequent contact with patients and their families.

5. Occupational therapists, physiotherapists and physiotherapists:
  - **Role:** They help with the rehabilitation and functional recovery of patients, working on mobility, strength, coordination or specific skills.
  - **Interaction:** They draw up rehabilitation plans in collaboration with neurologists and nurses, and provide regular feedback on patients' progress.

6. Neuropsychologists:
  - **Role:** They assess and treat cognitive, emotional and behavioural disorders associated with neurological conditions.
  - **Interaction:** They share their observations with the medical team and can suggest specific interventions or adaptations.

7. Social workers:
  - **Role:** They provide non-medical support, helping patients and their families to manage the social and financial aspects of the illness.
  - **Interaction:** They work with nurses and doctors to ensure that the patient's holistic needs are taken into account.

8. Pharmacists:
  - **Role:** They advise on medication and its side effects, and monitor drug interactions.
  - **Interactions:** They work in collaboration with the neurologists to optimise the medication regime and inform the nurses about the administration of the drugs.

The balance and effectiveness of this team is based on fluid communication and a mutual understanding of the roles and responsibilities of each member. Each member contributes to the team, and together they ensure that each patient receives comprehensive, personalised care. This inter-professional collaboration is the key to successful neurology treatment.

# Specialist neurology equipment

Neurology, as a medical discipline focused on the diagnosis, treatment and research of diseases of the nervous system, requires specialised equipment. This equipment provides precise information on the anatomy, physiology and pathology of the nervous system. Here is an overview of the key equipment used in this field:

1. Medical imaging:
   - **Computed tomography (CT):** Used to obtain detailed images of the brain and spinal cord, it is essential for detecting abnormalities such as tumours, bleeding or lesions.
   - **Magnetic resonance imaging (MRI):** Provides high-resolution images of nerve structures and is particularly useful for visualising lesions or demyelinating diseases such as multiple sclerosis.
   - **Positron emission tomography (PET):** Used in research and sometimes in clinical practice, PET measures the metabolic activity of the brain.
2. Clinical neurophysiology equipment:
   - **Electroencephalogram (EEG):** Measures the electrical activity of the brain, useful for diagnosing and monitoring conditions such as epilepsy.
   - **Electromyogram (EMG):** Assesses the electrical activity of muscles to diagnose neuromuscular disorders.
   - **Evoked potentials:** Measure the brain's electrical response to specific stimuli, enabling the function of certain nerve pathways to be assessed.

3. Intervention equipment:
  - **Surgical microscopes:** For delicate surgery on the nervous system.
  - **Deep brain stimulators:** Used to treat conditions such as Parkinson's disease.
  - **Thrombectomy equipment:** To remove blood clots in the event of a stroke.
4. Rehabilitation equipment:
  - **Treadmills with weight support:** Help patients regain mobility after a neurological injury.
  - **Rehabilitation robots:** Used to rehabilitate limbs after a stroke or other injury to the nervous system.
  - **Speech therapy equipment: For** speech and swallowing rehabilitation.
5. Monitoring and care equipment:
  - **Monitoring monitors:** For continuous monitoring of brain activity in intensive care unit patients.
  - **Programmable drug pumps:** For administering drugs directly into the cerebrospinal fluid or other areas of the body.
6. Search tools:
  - **Magnetoencephalography (MEG):** Measures the brain's magnetic activity, useful for pinpointing the origin of brain activity.
  - **Virtual reality equipment:** To study cognition and perception in a controlled environment.

Every piece of neurology equipment, whether for diagnosis, treatment or research, plays a vital role in furthering our understanding of the nervous system and improving patients' quality of life. Technology continues to evolve, offering ever more sophisticated possibilities for studying and treating neurological diseases.

# Chapter 3:
# THE FUNDAMENTAL SKILLS
# OF THE NEUROLOGY NURSE

## Neurological assessment :
## signs and symptoms

Neurological assessment is a systematic process designed to identify and interpret the signs and symptoms associated with disorders of the nervous system. It is crucial for making an accurate diagnosis and planning appropriate treatment. Signs are abnormalities detected during the physical examination, while symptoms are the sensations and problems reported by the patient.

1. Clinical interview:
This is the first stage of the assessment, in which the patient (or someone close to them) describes their medical history, current symptoms, their onset, duration and evolution, and any other relevant factors.
- **Common symptoms:** Headache, dizziness, vision problems, weakness, numbness, tremors, balance problems, difficulty speaking or swallowing, memory or behavioural problems.

2. Physical and neurological examination:
- **Mental evaluation:** Tests orientation, memory, attention, calculation and reasoning.
- **Cranial functions:** Examine pupils, eye movements, hearing, facial strength and sensation, taste, swallowing and facial expressions.
- **Muscular strength:** Check the strength of the different muscle groups in the limbs.
- **Sensation:** Testing tactile sensation, pain, temperature, vibration and proprioception.

- **Reflexes:** Test deep, superficial and plantar tendon reflexes.
- **Coordination:** Assessing the ability to perform rapid alternating movements and pointing-pointing tests.
- **Walking:** Observe the patient's gait, posture and ability to walk on their heels and toes, turn quickly, etc.

3. Specific signs and symptoms:
- **Hemiparesis:** Weakness on one side of the body.
- **Aphasia:** Difficulty in speaking or understanding language.
- **Ataxia:** Lack of coordination of movements.
- **Dysarthria:** Difficulty in articulating words.
- **Dysphagia:** Difficulty swallowing.
- **Nystagmus:** Involuntary, rhythmic eye movements.

4. Specialised tests:

These tests are carried out according to the patient's symptoms and may include blood tests, imaging studies (such as MRI or CT), EEG, EMG and other diagnostic tests to refine the diagnosis.

5. Assessment of associated systems:

It may be necessary to examine other body systems that can influence or be influenced by neurological disorders, such as the cardiovascular, musculoskeletal or endocrine systems.

Neurological assessment is a combination of medical art and science. It requires a methodical approach, careful observation and active listening. Neurological symptoms can often be subtle and vary considerably from one patient to another. Careful assessment allows us to make an accurate diagnosis, guide therapeutic interventions and evaluate the response to treatment.

# Care techniques specific to neurology

Caring for patients with neurological disorders is a unique challenge that requires specialist skills. Neurology nurses use a range of techniques to ensure optimal care for these patients. Let's take a closer look at these specialised techniques:

1. Ongoing neurological assessment:
Nurses must be trained to carry out targeted neurological examinations, regularly assessing the level of consciousness, motor skills, sensation, reflexes and function of the cranial nerves.

2. Intracranial management:
  - **Monitoring of intracranial pressure (ICP):** Involves the use of specialised devices to measure ICP in patients at risk.
  - **Techniques to reduce ICP:** Positioning, medication (such as mannitols), controlled hyperventilation, and sometimes surgery.

3. Crisis management:
  - **Continuous monitoring with EEG:** Enables early detection and treatment of seizures.
  - **Administration of anti-epileptic drugs:** Ensure appropriate doses and monitor for side effects.

4. Mobility management:
  - **Rehabilitation therapies:** Involve physiotherapy and occupational therapy to help recover function after neurological injury.
  - **Prevention of complications of immobility:** such as pressure sores, aspiration pneumonia and deep vein thrombosis.

5. Respiratory care:
    In patients with neurological disorders, it is crucial to keep the airway open and monitor respiratory function, particularly in those who are intubated or have swallowing problems.

6. Nutrition management:
- **Assessment of swallowing ability:** Before giving food or liquids.
- **Use of specialised feeding techniques:** such as feeding tubes or parenteral nutrition, for those who cannot swallow.

7. Appropriate communication:

Working with patients with speech or cognitive impairments requires the use of non-verbal communication methods, communication aids or validation techniques.

8. Patient and family education:

Informing patients and their families about the disease, prognosis, treatments and self-care techniques is essential. This can include demonstrations, discussions and written material.

9. Pain and comfort management:
- **Regular pain assessment:** Use appropriate pain scales.
- **Administration of analgesics:** As required and with monitoring of side effects.
- **Non-pharmacological techniques:** such as relaxation, distraction or physiotherapy.

10. Prevention of secondary complications:

Proactive care to prevent infections, cardiovascular complications, metabolic disorders and other complications associated with hospitalisation or the disease itself.

Neurology is a complex field that requires constant attention and specialist training to provide quality care. Neurology nurses play a pivotal role in patient management, using a combination of clinical, observational and communication skills to optimise outcomes for their patients.

# Managing pain and comfort

Pain management is at the heart of neurology nursing practice. Neurological, or neuropathic, pain is a complex pain resulting from injury or disease affecting the somatosensory nervous system. It differs from nociceptive pain, which is caused by tissue trauma. Proper management of this pain can significantly improve the patient's quality of life.

1. Understanding neurological pain:
    • **Characteristics:** Neuropathic pain is often described as burning, stabbing or electric shocks. It may be continuous or paroxysmal.
    • **Common causes:** Diabetic neuropathies, postherpetic neuralgia, post-stroke pain, HIV-associated neuropathies, multiple sclerosis, spinal cord injuries.
2. Pain assessment:
    • **Assessment tools:** Use standardised pain scales, such as the visual analogue scale (VAS) or the numerical intensity scale.
    • **Holistic assessment: Taking into account** the emotional, social and psychological factors that can influence the patient's perception of pain.
3. Pharmacological approaches:
    • **Tricyclic antidepressants (TCAs):** Such as amitriptyline, which has shown analgesic effects in certain neuropathies.
    • **Anticonvulsants:** Such as gabapentin and pregabalin, which are effective against several forms of neuropathic pain.
    • **Analgesics:** Opioids can be used, but with caution due to the risk of side effects and dependence.
    • **Lidocaine patches:** Can be used locally for localised pain.

4. Non-pharmacological techniques:
- **Transcutaneous electrical nerve stimulation (TENS):** A device that delivers small electrical currents to the skin to relieve pain.
- **Cognitive-behavioural therapies:** To help manage the psychological components of pain.
- **Relaxation and biofeedback:** To help relax the body and reduce muscle tension, which can amplify pain.
- **Acupuncture:** Some patients find relief with this age-old technique.

5. Comfort management:
- **Positioning:** Ensure a comfortable posture to reduce tension and pressure.
- **Massage:** Can help relax muscles and improve circulation.
- **Heat and cold:** Depending on the type of pain, hot or cold compresses may be beneficial.
- **Environment:** Maintain a calm environment, with soft lighting and an ambient temperature to help relaxation.

6. Patient education:
- **Understanding pain:** Helping patients to understand the nature of their pain.
- **Self-management strategies:** Include relaxation techniques, lifestyle modifications and recommendations for physical activity.
- **Drug side-effects:** Educating patients about potential side-effects and the importance of communication in adapting treatment.

Neurological pain can be difficult to treat and manage. A multimodal approach, combining pharmacological and non-pharmacological treatments, is often required. The role of the nurse is essential in assessing, treating and educating patients, to ensure optimal relief and improve their quality of life.

# Communication
# with a neurological patient

Communication is an essential element of care, and can be particularly complex when working with patients with neurological disorders. These patients may have cognitive, speech or comprehension deficits, making traditional communication difficult. The art of communicating effectively with them requires deep understanding, patience and appropriate strategies.

1. Understanding the specific challenges:
   - **Aphasia:** A disturbance in the ability to speak or understand language.
   - **Dysarthria:** Difficulty in articulating words due to muscular disorders.
   - **Cognitive:** Impaired memory, attention or decision-making.
   - **Sensory:** Hearing or vision problems that hinder communication.
2. Verbal methods:
   - **Speak slowly:** Give the patient time to process the information.
   - **Use simple language:** avoid medical jargon and keep sentences short.
   - **Repetition:** Repeat essential information to ensure understanding.
   - **Closed questions:** Using questions that require a 'yes' or 'no' answer may be easier for some patients.
3. Non-verbal methods:
   - **Gestures:** Use simple gestures to complete or replace words.
   - **Pictorial communication:** Using images, pictograms or drawings to facilitate understanding.

- **Lip-reading:** For patients who can lip-read, make sure you face the patient when speaking.
- **Writing:** Provide a board or tablet for the patient to write on.

4. Technological tools:
- **Communication applications:** Applications specially designed to facilitate communication with patients with speech deficits.
- **Tablets or computers:** With appropriate software to help with communication.

5. Adopting an active listening attitude:
- **Patience:** Giving the patient time to respond or express themselves.
- **Non-verbal feedback:** Use eye contact, head nods and facial expressions to show that you are listening and understand.
- **Clarification:** If you do not understand, politely ask the patient to repeat or explain in another way.

6. Involve informal carers:
- **Interpretation:** Family members or carers can often help interpret or explain the patient's needs.
- **Medical history:** This can provide essential information that the patient is unable to communicate.

7. Enabling environment:
- **Reduce noise:** A quiet environment makes it easier to concentrate and understand.
- **Adequate lighting:** Ensure there is good light for lip-reading or using visual methods.

8. Education and training:
- **Self-training:** Understanding the specifics of neurological disorders enables you to adapt your communication.
- **Further training:** Participating in specialist training courses or workshops on communicating with neurological patients.

Communicating with a neurological patient may require a different approach, but it remains a crucial element of care. By establishing effective communication, nurses can better understand the patient's needs, establish a climate of trust, and offer adapted, humanised care.

# Chapter 4:
# SUPPORT THE MAIN
# NEUROLOGICAL PATHOLOGIES

## Cerebrovascular accident (CVA)

### • Types and symptoms

A cerebrovascular accident (CVA), commonly known as a "stroke", is a medical emergency resulting from the interruption of blood flow to a part of the brain. This disruption may be due to blockage (ischaemia) or haemorrhage. Strokes are serious events that can result in lasting damage or even death.

1. Ischaemic stroke:
  • **Thrombotic:** Due to the formation of a blood clot (thrombus) in one of the arteries supplying the brain.
  • **Embolic:** A clot or other debris circulating in the blood (embolus) blocks a cerebral artery. These clots can form elsewhere in the body, often in the heart.

Symptoms:
  • Sudden paralysis or weakness of the face, arm or leg, usually on one side of the body.
  • Speech or comprehension problems.
  • Sudden loss of vision, particularly in one eye or on one side of the visual field.
  • Difficulty walking, dizziness, loss of balance or coordination.
  • Sudden, severe headaches with no known cause.

2. Haemorrhagic stroke:
  • **Intracerebral:** When the blood vessels in the brain burst, causing a haemorrhage into the surrounding brain tissue.

- **Subarachnoid:** Haemorrhage in the space between the brain and the surrounding membranes.

Symptoms:
- Sudden, intense headaches, often described as the "worst headaches" of the patient's life.
- Nausea and vomiting.
- Blurred or double vision.
- Light sensitivity.
- Loss of consciousness or confusion.
- Stiff neck.

3. Transient ischaemic attack (TIA):
- Often called a "mini-stroke", it is caused by a temporary interruption of blood flow to part of the brain. TIAs can last from a few minutes to several hours, but generally leave no lasting damage.

Symptoms:
- They are similar to those of an ischaemic stroke, but are temporary.
- Sudden weakness or numbness of the face, arm or leg.
- Sudden confusion, difficulty speaking or understanding.
- Sudden problems with sight or walking.
- Sudden dizziness or loss of balance.

When someone shows symptoms of stroke, it's essential to act quickly. Quick action can make the difference between a full recovery and lasting, even fatal, after-effects. The "FAST" (Face, Arms, Speech, Time) memory rule can help you recognise and react to a stroke: **Face** asymmetry, **Arm** weakness, Speech impairment and **Time to** call for help.

## • Nursing care

Caring for stroke patients is a complex process that requires a multidisciplinary approach. Nurses play an essential role at every stage of this process, from the moment the patient is admitted to hospital until they are discharged home or transferred to a rehabilitation facility. Here is an overview of the main nursing responsibilities and interventions in the care of stroke patients:

1. Initial assessment:
   - Monitoring vital signs and stabilisation.
   - Rapid neurological assessment: Glasgow score, pupillary reflexes, muscle strength, etc.
   - Collection of medical history and any medication, in particular anticoagulants.
2. Continuous monitoring:
   - Regular monitoring of neurological signs to detect any deterioration or improvement.
   - Monitoring vital parameters: blood pressure, heart rate, oxygen saturation.
   - Checking test results (brain scan, blood tests).
3. Airway management:
   - Ensuring the airways remain permeable.
   - Administration of oxygen if necessary.
   - Monitoring oxygen saturation and any signs of respiratory distress.
4. Nutrition and hydration management:
   - Assessment of swallowing before any oral intake to avoid false routes.
   - Placement of a nasogastric tube if necessary.
   - Monitoring fluid intake and output, maintaining hydration.
5. Mobilisation and prevention of complications:
   - Regular changes of position to prevent pressure sores.
   - Early mobilisation with the help of physiotherapists to reduce immobility.
   - Continence management: fitting urinary protection or catheters.
6. Pain management:
   - Regular pain assessment using appropriate scales.
   - Administration of painkillers as prescribed.

7. Education and support:
   - Inform patients and their families about the nature of the stroke, its after-effects and the prognosis.
   - Providing resources for rehabilitation and home support.
   - Encourage patients to take an active part in their rehabilitation.
8. Preparing for discharge:
   - Planning a return home or transfer to a rehabilitation centre.
   - Coordination with other healthcare professionals: physiotherapists, speech therapists, occupational therapists.
   - Ensuring continuity of care by providing recommendations and planning follow-up visits.

Nursing care for stroke patients requires a holistic, patient-centred approach. Nursing interventions aim to reduce complications, promote recovery and support the patient and family during this difficult period. Nurses' skill, empathy and dedication are essential to ensure optimal care for these patients.

# Epilepsy

## • Understanding epilepsy

Epilepsy is a neurological condition characterised by a predisposition to recurrent epileptic seizures. These seizures result from abnormal and excessive electrical activity in the brain. Although epilepsy is one of the oldest known medical conditions, many myths and misunderstandings persist about it. Let's find out more.

1. What is an epileptic seizure?
An epileptic seizure occurs when the normal electrical activity of the brain is suddenly disrupted. This can cause

changes in behaviour, sensation, movement and consciousness.

2. Classification of seizures:

- **Focal (or partial) seizures:** These begin in a specific region of the brain. They may be simple (without loss of consciousness) or complex (with altered consciousness).
- **Generalised seizures:** These affect both hemispheres of the brain from the outset. They include the following types: absence, myoclonic, tonic, atonic, clonic and tonic-clonic.

3. Causes of epilepsy:

- **Genetic origin:** Specific genetic mutations can make a person more susceptible to seizures.
- **Brain damage:** Trauma, stroke or infection of the brain (such as meningitis).
- **Congenital cerebral malformations:** Abnormalities in the development of the brain before birth.
- Metabolic or immunological disorders that may affect the brain.
- **Unknown factors:** In many cases, the exact cause remains undetermined.

4. Diagnosing epilepsy:

Diagnosis is based on a combination of tests, including clinical history, EEG (electroencephalogram) and sometimes brain imaging (MRI or CT scan).

5. Treatment:

- **Anti-epileptic drugs (AEDs):** These are the cornerstone of treatment. Their aim is to prevent seizures.
- **Surgery:** Indicated for certain people whose seizures are not controlled by medication and who have a localised area of the brain at the origin of the seizures.
- **Diets:** The ketogenic diet, rich in fats and low in carbohydrates, has shown beneficial effects in some patients.

- **Vagus nerve stimulation:** An approach that uses an implanted device to send electrical signals to the brain.

6. Living with epilepsy:
   - The challenges vary from person to person, but can include managing the side effects of medication, restrictions on certain activities and concerns about social stigma.
   - Awareness and education are essential to help people with epilepsy lead full and active lives.

7. Demystifying and raising awareness:
   - Epilepsy is not contagious.
   - An epileptic seizure is not always spectacular with convulsions; it can be manifested by a simple absence.
   - People with epilepsy can lead a normal life with the right treatment and support.

Understanding epilepsy is crucial not only for people with the condition and their families, but also for society as a whole. Better knowledge of the condition can foster empathy, awareness and better support for those living with epilepsy.

## • Crisis management

Seizure management is essential to ensure patient safety, minimise potential injury and provide appropriate support. It requires a clear understanding of what to expect during a seizure and what action to take.

1. Recognition of the crisis:
   - Understand the warning signs or 'auras' that some people may experience.
   - Identify the different types of crisis so that you can intervene appropriately.

2. Putting safety first:
- Move the patient away from any potential hazards (sharp objects, hard corners, stairs).
- Place the patient in the lateral safety position to avoid aspiration of secretions and to facilitate breathing.
- Protect your head with a cushion or jacket to avoid trauma.
- Do not attempt to restrain the patient or limit their movements.
- Do not insert anything into the patient's mouth.
3. Surveillance:
- Note the duration of the seizure. If a seizure lasts longer than 5 minutes or if a second seizure occurs immediately after the first, emergency medical assistance is required.
- Observe the characteristics of the seizure to inform medical staff: type of movements, duration, loss of consciousness, tongue biting, etc.
4. After the crisis:
- Keep the patient in the lateral safety position until they recover.
- Be reassuring and calm when the person comes to; they may be disorientated or confused.
- Avoid giving food or drink until the person has fully recovered.
- Inform the patient of what has happened in a clear and simple manner.
5. How to prepare:
- If you are in regular contact with someone who has epilepsy, always have a seizure plan to hand.
- Be aware of any emergency medication the person may need.
6. Education:
- Make sure that family members, teachers, colleagues and friends of the person with epilepsy know about first aid in the event of a seizure.
- Ask the person with epilepsy or their family if there are any specific measures they should take.

7. When to consult immediately:
- If the seizure lasts longer than 5 minutes.
- If another crisis starts shortly after the first.
- If the person does not regain consciousness after the seizure.
- If the person is injured during the seizure.
- If the person has persistent difficulty breathing after the attack.

Managing epileptic seizures requires calm, quick decision-making and caring attention. With the right knowledge and preparation, the risks associated with an epileptic seizure can be significantly reduced, ensuring the safety and well-being of the patient.

# Degenerative diseases (e.g. Parkinson's, Alzheimer's)

## · Features and challenges

Degenerative diseases are characterised by a progressive deterioration in the structures or functions of cells, tissues or organs. These diseases, which mainly affect the nervous system, represent a major challenge for patients, their families and healthcare professionals.

1. Characteristics of degenerative diseases:
- **Slow but steady progression:** Although the rate of progression varies from disease to disease, deterioration is generally inexorable.
- **Neurological damage:** These diseases often affect the nervous system, which can lead to motor, cognitive, sensory or behavioural symptoms.
- **Multifactorial origin:** They may result from a combination of genetic, environmental and metabolic factors.

2. Examples of degenerative diseases:
  - **Alzheimer's disease:** Characterised by a progressive loss of memory and other cognitive functions.
  - **Parkinson's disease:** Manifested mainly by tremors, muscular rigidity and bradykinesia.
  - **Amyotrophic lateral sclerosis (ALS):** A disease that affects motor neurons, leading to progressive paralysis.
3. Challenges posed by degenerative diseases:
  - **Early diagnosis:** Many of these diseases have no specific signs at onset, making early diagnosis difficult.
  - **Treatment:** To date, there is often no cure for these diseases, only symptomatic treatments.
  - **Emotional burden:** The inevitable progression of the disease can be devastating for patients and their families.
  - **Care needs:** As the disease progresses, the patient may require increased assistance, ranging from home help to admission to specialised institutions.
  - **Economic cost:** The cost of care and treatment can be high, putting a strain on healthcare systems and families.
  - **Research: Although there have been** advances, research into these diseases is complex, requiring multidisciplinary resources and collaboration.
  - **Raising awareness: There is** a constant need to educate the public and healthcare professionals about these diseases, their symptoms and best management practices.
4. Comprehensive care:
  - **Multidisciplinary approach:** Optimal patient care often requires the involvement of neurologists, physiotherapists, speech therapists and social workers, among others.

- **Psychological support:** Psychological support is essential for patients and their families, given the emotional challenges that these illnesses impose.
- **Rehabilitation:** Rehabilitation programmes can help maintain a patient's independence for as long as possible.

Degenerative diseases, with their inexorable progression and profound impact on daily life, represent a colossal challenge. However, thanks to medical innovation, research and multidisciplinary care, significant improvements in patients' quality of life are possible.

## • Specific support and care

Patients suffering from degenerative diseases require special attention and care tailored to their condition. The progressive nature of these diseases requires a proactive approach, combining medical care, rehabilitation and psychosocial support.

1. Full assessment:
   - **Medical assessment:** To determine the stage of the disease, identify any complications and adapt the treatment.
   - **Functional assessment:** To assess the patient's abilities and limitations in activities of daily living.
   - **Psychological assessment:** To identify symptoms such as depression, anxiety or other mood disorders.
2. Therapeutic interventions:
   - **Medication:** Medication can help manage some symptoms, although its effectiveness varies from person to person.
   - **Physical therapy:** To maintain mobility, strengthen muscles and prevent contractures.

- **Occupational therapy:** To help patients adapt their daily activities and maintain their independence for as long as possible.
- **Speech therapy: Particularly** for patients with speech or swallowing difficulties.

3. Psychosocial support:
- **Individual therapy:** To help the patient manage stress, anxiety and emotions linked to the illness.
- **Support groups:** These provide a space where patients and their families can share their experiences and get mutual support.
- **Family counselling:** To help family members understand the disease, manage the associated stress and provide the best possible care.

4. Home adaptations:
- **Technical aids:** such as wheelchairs, medical beds, grab bars and other devices to facilitate mobility.
- **Home modifications:** Making the house accessible, such as installing ramps, widening doorways or modifying bathrooms.

5. Communication support:
- **Assistive devices:** For patients with speech difficulties, such as voice synthesizers.
- **Communication therapy:** To develop strategies and skills to compensate for the loss of verbal functions.

6. Long-term planning:
- **Palliative care:** To manage pain and other uncomfortable symptoms, and to provide emotional and spiritual support.
- **Advance directives:** Encouraging patients to express their wishes regarding future care, resuscitation or other medical interventions.

7. Education and training:
- **For patients:** helping them to understand their illness, the treatments available and how to manage their symptoms.

- **For families and carers:** To provide tools and strategies for caring effectively for the patient while preserving their own well-being.

Caring for patients with degenerative diseases requires a holistic approach that goes beyond simple medical treatment. It requires close collaboration between patients, their families, healthcare professionals and other stakeholders to ensure optimal quality of life despite the progression of the disease.

# Chapter 5:
# EMERGENCY SITUATIONS IN NEUROLOGY

## Recognising a neurological emergency

One of the fundamental aspects of the neurology nurse's role is the ability to quickly identify a neurological emergency. These emergencies, if not treated immediately, can result in permanent damage to the brain or other parts of the nervous system. Here are the signs, symptoms and conditions that require immediate intervention:

**1. Signs of a stroke:**
Known by the acronym "FAST":
- **F (Face)** : Asymmetry of the face, for example, if one side of the face sags when the person is asked to smile.
- **A (Arms)**: Weakness or numbness in one arm. If one arm drops when the person is asked to raise both arms, this is a warning sign.
- **S (Speech)**: Difficulty speaking or unintelligible speech.
- **T (Time)**: It is crucial to act quickly in the event of a suspected stroke.

**2. Prolonged epileptic seizure:**
Any seizure lasting more than 5 minutes or consecutive seizures without regaining consciousness between them.

**3. Head trauma:**
Especially if it is associated with loss of consciousness, vomiting, intense headaches or a change in behaviour.

**4. Sudden or severe increase in intracranial pressure:**
Symptoms such as intense headaches, nausea, vomiting, reduced consciousness or a change in the size or reactivity of the pupils.

**5. Meningitis:**
Symptoms include fever, stiff neck, photophobia (sensitivity to light), **intense** headaches **and sometimes skin rashes.**

**6. Guillain-Barré syndrome:**
Ascending paralysis that generally begins in the feet and legs and moves upwards, associated with numbness or weakness.

**7. Compression of the spinal cord:**
May manifest as sudden weakness, paralysis, loss of sensation or bladder or bowel problems.

**8. Impaired vision:**
Sudden loss of vision, double vision or severe eye pain may indicate conditions such as optic neuritis or acute glaucoma.

**9. Severe migraine:**
Especially if it differs from previous episodes or is accompanied by focal neurological symptoms.

**10. Sudden alteration in consciousness:**
This can be due to a variety of causes, from hypoglycaemia (low blood sugar) to a brain tumour.

Every second counts in neurology. If a patient presents with any of the above symptoms or signs, it is essential to seek immediate medical attention. Neurology nurses are often the first to recognise these signs and initiate rapid intervention, playing a vital role in limiting potential damage and maximising patient outcomes.

# Nursing intervention in an emergency

Neurological emergencies can occur at any time and require a rapid, structured and coordinated response from healthcare professionals, including nurses. These delicate situations require not only clinical skills but also the ability to manage stress and communicate effectively with the medical team and the patient's family. Here is an overview of nursing intervention in neurological emergencies:

1. Initial assessment:
- **ABC (Airway, Breathing, Circulation)**: Ensure airway is clear, check breathing and circulation.
- **Measurement of vital signs:** heart rate, blood pressure, respiratory rate, oxygen saturation.
- **Level of consciousness:** Use of the Glasgow Scale to assess the level of consciousness.
- **Rapid neurological examination:** pupil reactivity, limb movements, response to stimuli.

2. Alert and communication:
- Immediately inform the doctor or emergency team of the patient's condition.
- Use effective communication methods such as SBAR (Situation, Background, Assessment, Recommendation) to convey clear and precise information.

3. Patient stabilisation:
- Position the patient safely, for example in a lateral decubitus position in the event of an epileptic seizure.
- Ensure adequate oxygenation, in particular by administering oxygen if necessary.
- Prepare the equipment needed for intubation or other urgent interventions.

4. Continuous monitoring:
- Regular monitoring of vital signs and neurological status.
- Monitor for complications such as cerebral oedema, hernia, hypoxia, etc.
- Document all changes and interventions.

5. Medication:
- Rapidly administer medicines prescribed in emergency situations, such as anticonvulsants in the event of an epileptic seizure.
- Prepare administration routes, such as a peripheral venous line.

6. Emotional support:
- Reassure the patient, even if they are unconscious. Touch, words and presence can be soothing.
- Inform and support the family, explaining the situation and the measures taken.

7. Preparation for examinations or interventions:
- Preparing the patient for diagnostic tests such as MRI, CT scan, lumbar puncture, etc.
- Assisting the medical team during procedures such as the insertion of a ventricular drainage catheter.

8. Education:
- Once the situation has stabilised, educate the patient and family about what has happened, the possible causes and the steps to be taken.

9. Post-emergency debriefing:
- Discussing events with the team, analysing the emergency response and identifying areas for improvement.

Intervening in neurological emergencies requires sharp skills, rapid judgement and the ability to work as part of a team. Nurses play a crucial role in the early recognition of emergency signs, initiating intervention, stabilising the patient and providing emotional support to patients and their families.

## Working with the medical team

In neurology, a multidisciplinary approach is essential. Neurological patients can present with a range of complex symptoms that require the expertise of a variety of health professionals. The neurology nurse is an essential link in this team. Here's a look at how nurses work with the neurology medical team:

1. The nurse and the neurologist:
   - **Ongoing communication**: The nurse communicates daily observations, changes in the patient's condition and responses to treatment to the neurologist.
   - **Care planning**: Nurses play an active role in creating and implementing the care plan, taking account of the neurologist's recommendations.
2. Collaboration with the neurosurgeon:
   - **Pre-operative preparation**: The nurse prepares the patient for surgery, ensures that all the necessary tests are carried out, and educates the patient about what to expect.
   - **Post-operative care**: After surgery, the nurse monitors the patient closely for possible complications and ensures that pain is well managed.
3. Work with the neuropsychologist:
   - Neuropsychologists assess and treat cognitive deficits. The nurse can provide valuable information about the patient's day-to-day behaviour, challenges and progress.
4. Interaction with physiotherapists and occupational therapists:
   - These therapists work on mobility, strength and daily activities. The nurse coordinates with them to ensure that the patient is ready for therapy and to discuss any progress or problems encountered.
5. Collaboration with speech therapists:
   - For patients with speech or swallowing difficulties, the nurse collaborates with the speech therapist, sharing observations and implementing food safety recommendations.

6. Coordination with social workers and psychologists:
- These professionals help patients and their families to manage emotional stress, plan for discharge and access resources. The nurse informs them of the psychosocial needs of the patient and their family.

7. Communication with radiology and laboratory technicians:
- The nurse ensures that patients are prepared for examinations, that samples are correctly taken and transmitted, and that the results are communicated to the appropriate team.

8. Exchanges with pharmacists:
- The nurse discusses patients' medication regimes, potential interactions and side effects with pharmacists to ensure safe and effective use of medicines.

Neurology is a field where the complexity of cases requires close collaboration between different professionals. The nurse, as the pivot of care, plays a central role in coordinating and communicating within this team. This collaboration guarantees comprehensive, individualised patient care, optimising results and improving the quality of care.

# Chapter 6:
# EMOTIONAL CHALLENGES
# AND PSYCHOLOGICAL

## Understanding the psychological repercussions of neurological disorders

Neurological conditions are not limited to physical and cognitive symptoms. They often have a profound impact on patients' mental and emotional health. Understanding and addressing these psychological impacts is essential to providing holistic care. Here is a detailed overview of these consequences and how to manage them.

1. Acceptance of the diagnosis:
   - **Shock and denial**: The initial diagnosis of a neurological condition can be overwhelming, leading to initial denial.
   - **Anger and frustration**: With realisation, anger and frustration often arise, linked to the question "Why me?
   - **Negotiation**: Some people may try to 'negotiate' their health, hoping for respite or a cure.
   - **Depression**: Sadness, despair and a sense of isolation can arise from understanding the extent and chronicity of the illness.
   - **Acceptance**: With time and support, many patients come to terms with their condition, although this is not a linear process.
2. Modified identity management:
   - **Loss of independence**: Physical or cognitive limitations can make it difficult to carry out daily tasks, impacting on the patient's autonomy.

- **Role modification**: Patients may feel that they can no longer fulfil their previous role as a parent, partner or professional.
- **Self-esteem**: Increased dependence can lead to low self-esteem and feelings of worthlessness.

3. Impact on relationships:
- **Social isolation:** Communication challenges, reduced mobility or fear of embarrassment can lead to social withdrawal.
- **Relationship strain**: Carers and family members can also be stressed, leading to relationship strain.

4. Anxiety and depression:
- **Fear of progression**: Uncertainty about the course of the disease can be a constant source of anxiety.
- **Somatic symptoms**: Depression can also manifest itself through physical symptoms, such as headaches or pain, further complicating the clinical picture.

5. Cognitive and emotional issues:
- **Cognitive frustration**: Difficulty concentrating, remembering or processing information can be a source of frustration.
- **Emotional lability**: Certain neurological conditions can cause rapid fluctuations in mood or inappropriate emotional responses.

Management and support:
- **Therapy**: Psychotherapy can help patients deal with their emotions, develop coping strategies and improve their quality of life.
- **Support groups**: Support groups provide a platform for sharing experiences and getting advice.
- **Medication**: In some cases, medication to treat anxiety or depression may be beneficial.
- **Education**: Understanding the disease can help reduce anxiety and make you feel more in control.

Neurological conditions have a profound impact not only on the body but also on the mind. As carers, it is crucial to recognise these psychological repercussions and offer appropriate support, thereby ensuring that patients receive comprehensive care.

# The importance of active listening

Active listening is an essential skill for any healthcare professional. In neurology, where patients may face communication challenges or profound upheavals in their lives, this skill becomes even more crucial. Let's delve into the importance of active listening in this particular field.

1. Humanising care:
   - **Recognition of the individual**: Beyond their diagnosis, each patient is a person with a history, emotions and concerns. Active listening helps to recognise and validate this individuality.
   - **Dignity and respect**: By taking the time to listen attentively, the nurse confers on the patient the dignity and respect essential to a quality therapeutic relationship.
2. Improved clinical understanding:
   - **Nuanced details**: By listening actively, the nurse can pick up nuances or details that might be missed in one-way communication.
   - **Comprehensive assessment**: Neurological symptoms can be subtle or complex. Active listening provides a complete picture of the patient's challenges.
3. Facilitating communication:
   - **Encouraging expression**: Patients with neurological conditions may have difficulty communicating. Active listening encourages patients to express themselves in the knowledge that they are being heard.

- **Clarification**: By reflecting and asking questions, the nurse can clarify and confirm understanding of the information shared.

4. Establishing trust:
- **Emotional safety**: Patients are more likely to share deep concerns or fears if they feel listened to and validated.
- **Therapeutic relationship**: Mutual trust is essential for an effective carer-patient relationship. Active listening lays the foundations for this trust.

5. Managing emotions:
- **Comfort**: For many patients, simply being listened to can offer great comfort in the face of anxiety or distress.
- **Patient advocacy**: By deeply understanding the patient's concerns and needs, the nurse is better equipped to advocate for appropriate interventions or care.

6. Education and advice:
- **Identifying information needs**: By listening actively, the nurse can identify areas where the patient needs further information or clarification.
- **Targeted guidance**: Advice or education can be tailored to the patient's specific concerns, making guidance more relevant and effective.

Active listening is not just a communication skill; it is fundamental to the delivery of quality care. In neurology, where the challenges are multiple and complex, taking the time to truly listen can make all the difference in a patient's life.

## Managing stress and burnout

In neurology, as in many medical fields, healthcare professionals are faced with particularly demanding and intense situations. The complexity of cases, the emotional distress of patients and their families, and the workload can quickly become sources of accumulated stress. If this stress is not properly managed, it can lead to burnout, a state of emotional, physical and mental exhaustion.

Working in neurology requires a depth of knowledge, technical dexterity and an ability to navigate the tumultuous waters of human emotions. Every day, nurses and doctors witness triumphs and tragedies, remarkable recoveries and inevitable setbacks. These experiences, while deeply gratifying, are also a source of emotional strain.

The key is early recognition of the signs of stress and burnout. Persistent feelings of fatigue, cynicism, detachment from patients, reduced capacity for empathy, or feelings of ineffectiveness at work are all warning signs. Ignoring these signs can lead not only to a deterioration in the quality of care, but also to health problems for the carer themselves.

Managing stress involves adopting both personal and professional strategies. On a personal level, it is crucial to maintain a balance between work and private life. This can mean making time for hobbies, family or relaxing activities such as meditation or sport. It's also important to eat a balanced diet, get enough sleep and seek support when needed, whether from loved ones, colleagues or mental health professionals.

At work, setting clear boundaries, taking regular breaks and attending training courses or workshops on stress management can be beneficial. Talking to colleagues, taking part in support groups or simply sharing experiences can also help to put things into perspective and provide strategies for coping with everyday challenges.

Above all, we need to remember that asking for help is not a sign of weakness. In a world where self-sacrifice is often seen as a virtue, recognising your own needs and limitations is in fact an act of strength. After all, taking care of ourselves is an essential first step to being able to take care of others.

Neurology, with all its challenges, is also a field of profound humanity and gratification. By protecting themselves from burnout, healthcare professionals can continue to offer quality care to those who need it most.

# Chapter 7:
# PHARMACOLOGY
# SPECIFIC TO NEUROLOGY

## Overview of medicines commonly used

In neurology, a variety of drugs are used to treat, manage and relieve the symptoms of neurological disorders. These drugs, which are specially designed to target and act on the nervous system, are essential for ensuring patients' quality of life.

Diseases of the brain and nervous system are complex, and the medicines used reflect this complexity. Often, a patient may require a combination of drugs, adjusted according to individual needs.

**1. Anti-epileptics:** Used mainly to treat epilepsy, these drugs help to control and prevent seizures. Common examples include carbamazepine, valproate, lamotrigine and levetiracetam.

**2. Dopamine modulators:** Prescribed mainly for Parkinson's disease, these drugs act by altering the levels of dopamine in the brain. Levodopa is a classic example, often combined with carbidopa to increase its effectiveness.

**3. Anti-Alzheimer's drugs:** These work by slowing the progression of Alzheimer's symptoms. Donepezil, rivastigmine and memantine are among the most commonly prescribed.

**4. Antispastic drugs:** For patients with multiple sclerosis or other conditions that cause muscle spasms, drugs such as baclofen and tizanidine are often used.

**5. Anti-migraine drugs:** For migraine sufferers, there is a range of drugs, including triptans such as sumatriptan, which help to reduce the frequency and severity of attacks.

**6. Immunosuppressants:** These drugs, such as natalizumab and fingolimod, are used in the treatment of multiple sclerosis to modulate the activity of the immune system.

**7. Anticoagulants and antiplatelet agents:** For patients who have suffered a stroke or are at risk, these drugs help prevent the formation of blood clots. Aspirin, clopidogrel and warfarin are common examples.

**8. Neuromodulators:** To treat conditions such as neuropathy or fibromyalgia, neuromodulators such as gabapentin and pregabalin are commonly prescribed.

**9. Cholinergic agents:** These are used to treat movement disorders, such as myasthenia gravis, by increasing the activity of the neurotransmitter acetylcholine.

**10. Antivertigo drugs:** For patients suffering from vertigo or illnesses such as Meniere's disease, drugs such as betahistine may be prescribed.

Knowledge of these drugs, their side effects and interactions is crucial for any professional working in neurology. Each drug has its own specificities, and an individualised approach is often necessary to ensure the best therapeutic outcome for the patient. This list is only an outline of commonly used drugs, highlighting the depth and diversity of treatments available in the vast field of neurology.

# Administration, side effects and interactions

In the complex field of neurology, mastery of drug administration, as well as knowledge of possible side effects and interactions, is essential to ensure the safety and efficacy of treatment.

## 1. Administration :
The way in which a medicine is administered can influence its effectiveness. For example, some drugs are taken on an empty stomach, while others must be taken with food. In addition, some neurological drugs are administered orally, others by injection, and still others may need to be administered intrathecally (into the cerebrospinal fluid).

- **Oral route:** Tablets, capsules and syrups are the most common forms. It is essential to follow the prescribed doses and times of administration to ensure the effectiveness and safety of the treatment.
- **Injection:** Some medicines, such as immunomodulators, may need to be administered by injection, whether subcutaneously, intramuscularly or intravenously.
- **Other routes:** Devices such as baclofen pumps administer the drug directly into the cerebrospinal fluid.
- 

## 2. Side effects :
Almost all medicines can cause side effects. In neurology, these effects can range from mild to severe.

- **Mild:** Fatigue, dizziness, gastrointestinal problems, headaches, dry mouth.
- **Moderate:** Trembling, weight gain, cognitive impairment, vision problems.
- **Serious:** Allergic reactions, respiratory depression, cardiac problems, hepatotoxicity.

It is crucial for nurses and doctors to monitor these side effects and inform patients of what they need to watch out for.

**3. Interactions :**
Many neurological patients may be taking several medications, which increases the risk of drug interactions.

- **Drug-drug:** For example, combining anti-epileptic drugs with certain antibiotics can reduce the effectiveness of the anti-epileptic drugs.
- **Food and medication:** Eating grapefruit, for example, can interact with certain neurological drugs and affect their metabolism.
- **Drug-affected:** Patients with certain medical conditions, such as renal or hepatic impairment, may have a different or exacerbated response to certain drugs.

Managing medicines in neurology is a delicate task that requires constant attention and in-depth knowledge. Nurses play a crucial role in educating patients, monitoring side effects and ensuring that medicines are administered correctly. Close collaboration between members of the care team is also essential to ensure patient safety and well-being.

# The importance of drug adherence in neurology

In the dynamic and complex field of neurology, medication adherence is of paramount importance. This chapter highlights why it is vital that patients adhere strictly to their medication regime and how nurses can play a crucial role in facilitating this adherence.

Neurology is a branch of medicine concerned with the diagnosis and treatment of disorders of the nervous system, which are often chronic and require long-term drug management. In this context, adherence to medication is more crucial than ever. Not only does it improve symptom control, it can also prevent the progression of disease and reduce the risk of complications.

## The Components of Drug Adhesion
1. Understanding the disease :
Above all, patients need to understand the nature of their illness and the reason for the medication prescribed. A thorough understanding helps to create a sense of responsibility and of taking active charge of their health.
2. Medication Routine :
Establishing a stable medication routine is vital. This may involve the use of pillboxes, alarms or smartphone apps that remind patients to take their medication at specific times.
3. Managing side effects :
Side effects are one of the main reasons for non-adherence. By working closely with doctors, nurses can help adjust doses or types of medication to minimise these undesirable effects.

## The role of the nurse
1. Education and information :
Nurses are responsible for informing patients about the importance of adherence, providing them with detailed information about medicines, including the correct way to take them and potential side effects.
2. Emotional Support :
Nurses must also offer emotional support, encouraging patients to express their concerns and helping them to manage the anxiety or depression that can accompany neurological conditions.
3. Multidisciplinary collaboration :
Nurses need to work closely with the whole medical team, including doctors, pharmacists and social workers, to develop and implement effective medication adherence strategies.

<u>4. Regular monitoring :</u>
Nurses play a crucial role in the regular monitoring of medication adherence, continually assessing the effectiveness of the medication regime and adjusting care plans accordingly.

In the ongoing journey of managing neurological disorders, adherence to medication is a guiding star, guiding patients towards a better quality of life. Nurses, with their skill and compassion, are pillars in achieving this goal, facilitating the path to better health and lasting wellbeing for their patients.

# Chapter 8:
# THE RELATIONSHIP WITH THE FAMILY AND CARERS

## Understanding the role of carers in care

The care pathway for a patient with neurological disorders, or other chronic conditions, is a multifaceted process that is not limited to the patient-healthcare professional relationship. An often overlooked but essential player in this equation is the carer. These individuals, whether family members, friends or professionals, play a pivotal role in the patient's day-to-day support.

**The Faces of Caring**
A carer is not always easy to identify. They may be a spouse who accompanies their partner to medical appointments, a child who cares for an elderly parent, or even a friend who helps a relative manage their medication. In some cases, carers are professionals, such as home carers, who provide care in the home.

The Multiple Roles of the Carer
- **Emotional support:** Faced with illness, uncertainty and fear can be overwhelming. The carer provides constant emotional support, comforting the patient and helping them to cope with the challenges.
- **Day-to-day assistance:** For many patients, everyday tasks can become difficult. The carer can help with meal preparation, washing, getting around and other day-to-day needs.
- **Managing medication:** The carer ensures that medication is taken correctly and on time, and can also help to recognise and manage any side effects.

- **Liaison with healthcare professionals:** The carer often acts as an intermediary between the patient and their medical team, helping to communicate concerns, understand medical instructions and follow care plans.
- **Logistical support:** This includes coordinating medical appointments, transport and, if necessary, managing the financial or administrative aspects of care.

### The Challenges of Caring

Being a carer is no easy task. The emotional and physical burden can be heavy. They can feel tired, stressed and even burnt out. Recognising their needs is therefore essential. It's important that they have access to resources, such as support groups or training, to help them in their role.

### The Importance of Recognition

Recognising the value of carers in the care process is crucial. Healthcare professionals need to work closely with them, seeing them as partners in the patient's care. Open and respectful communication is essential.

In the complex and often tumultuous landscape of healthcare, the carer stands like a beacon, illuminating and securing the path for the patient. By understanding and valuing their role, we can better serve not only patients, but also those who support them with such dedication and love.

# Effective communication with the family

Communication is one of the pillars of care, and when it comes to treating patients with neurological disorders or other complex pathologies, it does not stop at the relationship between the healthcare professional and the patient. It is just as crucial to communicate effectively with the family. The family is often the patient's main emotional and practical support, and is deeply invested in the patient's well-being. The way in which carers interact with the family can greatly influence the healing process, as well as the emotional and psychological well-being of all involved.

In the vast ecosystem of healthcare, the family occupies a central place. They are the patient's memory when he cannot express himself, they are the guardians of his wishes and desires, and they are often the ones who keep a watchful eye on the slightest changes in his condition. Yet it is also made up of individuals with their own concerns, their own hopes and their own needs for information.

The key to effective communication with the family lies in empathy and listening. It's not enough to inform; you also have to understand. Families are immersed in a complex medical world that they don't always understand. Every machine, every medical term and every new treatment can seem intimidating. Carers, with their expertise, have a responsibility to decipher this world for them, not by oversimplifying, but by illuminating with patience and compassion.

It's also important to remember that every family is unique. Some may need in-depth details to feel involved and reassured, while others may feel overwhelmed by too much information. Some may want to be actively involved in care, while others may prefer to stand back. The art of communication lies in the ability to read these individual needs and adapt accordingly.

It is also essential to provide a space where families can ask questions, express concerns or simply share their emotions. These exchanges should not only occur at crises or key decision points, but should be encouraged throughout the care process.

Ultimately, effective communication with the family transcends mere words. It is rooted in mutual respect, understanding and a sincere desire to accompany the patient and their loved ones through the labyrinth of medical care. It requires not only skill, but also heart, providing a bridge between medical science and the shared humanity that binds us all.

## Supporting carers in the face of challenges neurological disease

Behind every patient with a neurological disease, there is often a constellation of carers - individuals who offer support, care and love. These caregivers, whether parents, spouses, friends or professionals, become a silent but powerful force in the patient's journey. However, the challenges of neurological disease not only affect the patient, they also profoundly shape the lives of these carers. Supporting these carers is an essential step in ensuring effective overall care.

Neurological disease, with its spectrum of symptoms ranging from physical pain to mental confusion, can be a mountain to climb not only for the patient, but also for the carer. Watching a loved one struggle with the disease can be heartbreaking, and the workload for the carer can be exhausting. However, just as illness presents challenges, it also offers the opportunity to forge deeper bonds, cultivate patience, and discover unsuspected reserves of resilience.

## Understanding Pressures on the Carer

As well as playing a key role in supporting the patient, carers face multiple pressures. There is the emotional pressure of seeing a loved one suffer, the physical pressure of daily care and the psychological pressure of always being 'on the alert', anticipating needs and responding to crises.

## Providing emotional support

It is crucial to recognise the emotional impact that caring for someone with a neurological condition can have. Carers need spaces to express their emotions, whether through support groups, individual therapy or simply honest conversations with loved ones.

## Providing Resources and Training

Carers, especially if they are new to the role, can feel at a loss when faced with the demands of care. Providing training on how to manage certain symptoms, use equipment or communicate effectively can be a real lifeline.

## Stressing the Importance of Rest

Caregiver burnout is real. Just as patients need care, carers need rest. It is essential to encourage carers to take time out for themselves, whether to relax, do something they enjoy or simply rest.

## Create a Community

Carers need to know that they are not alone. Connecting them to a community of others in similar situations can provide an invaluable support network. They can share advice, stories and resources, or simply offer a listening ear.

Caring for those who care for others is an essential part of managing neurological diseases. By supporting these carers, we strengthen the chain of care that surrounds each patient, ensuring a better quality of life for all.

# Chapter 9:
# REHABILITATION
# AND REHABILITATION IN NEUROLOGY

## Basic principles
## neurological rehabilitation

Neurological rehabilitation is a medical discipline that aims to improve and restore the functions of individuals suffering from neurological disorders. Using a multidisciplinary approach, it aims to help patients regain an optimal level of independence in their daily activities. The basic principles of neurological rehabilitation are based on an in-depth understanding of the nervous system and its ability to repair, adapt and reconfigure itself.

### 1. Brain Plasticity
One of the fundamental principles of neurological rehabilitation is brain plasticity. This is the ability of the nervous system to reorganise itself in response to injury. This reorganisation can be stimulated by specific therapies, encouraging the recovery of lost functions.

### 2. Customised approach
Each individual is unique, as are the neurological injuries or illnesses they may suffer. Consequently, rehabilitation must be individualised, based on the patient's needs, abilities and goals.

### 3. Early intervention
Early treatment is often associated with better results. Starting rehabilitation soon after an injury or the onset of a disease can maximise the benefits of brain plasticity and minimise secondary complications.

## 4. Multidisciplinary approach

Neurological rehabilitation involves a team of professionals, including neurologists, physiotherapists, occupational therapists, speech therapists, neuropsychologists and other specialists. Each member brings his or her own expertise to bear on the multidimensional challenges associated with neurological conditions.

## 5. Education and empowerment

It is essential that patients and their families understand the nature of the illness or injury, as well as the aims of rehabilitation. Education empowers patients and their families, enabling them to make informed decisions and play an active part in the recovery process.

## 6. Continuous reassessment

The rehabilitation process requires constant evaluation and reassessment. As the patient progresses, objectives and interventions may need to be adjusted.

## 7. Holistic approach

In addition to physical interventions, it is equally crucial to take care of the emotional, psychological and social aspects of the patient. Healing and rehabilitation encompass the whole person.

## 8. Promoting activity and participation

Encouraging patients to play an active role in the rehabilitation process not only enhances physical recovery, but also boosts self-esteem and confidence.

## 9. Adapted environment

A suitable and stimulating environment is crucial. Specific facilities and equipment can help maximise the results of rehabilitation.

## 10. Social integration

One of the main objectives is to reintegrate the patient into society. This may mean returning to work, resuming recreational activities, or simply being able to interact socially.

Neurological rehabilitation is a process
It is a complex and dynamic condition that requires a coordinated, patient and detailed approach to restore function and improve quality of life.

# Working with therapists (physiotherapy, speech therapy, etc.)

Caring for a neurology patient does not rely solely on nursing or medical care. It requires a holistic approach, integrating various therapeutic specialities. Close collaboration between nurses and therapists, such as physiotherapists, speech therapists, occupational therapists and others, is crucial to ensuring complete and effective rehabilitation. Let's take a look at how this collaboration works on a day-to-day basis, and how it contributes to optimal patient care.

**1. Open and Regular Communication**
At the heart of any successful collaboration is transparent communication. Nurses and therapists need to communicate regularly about the patient's condition, treatment goals and progress. This can take the form of team meetings, notes in the patient's medical file, or informal discussions.

**2. Understanding Roles**
Each professional brings a unique expertise to the rehabilitation process. The nurse may have an overall perspective of the patient's condition, while the physiotherapist focuses on mobility, the speech therapist on speech and swallowing, and so **on. Understanding each person's role enables the patient to be directed to the right specialist at the right time.**

**3. Setting common objectives**
Setting the patient's goals is often a collective effort. Nurses, with their in-depth knowledge of the patient, can

help to establish realistic and appropriate objectives, in collaboration with the therapists.

## 4. Cross Support

Nurses can reinforce therapists' interventions by reminding patients of their physiotherapy exercises, monitoring safety during occupational therapy sessions, or helping with techniques learned in speech therapy. Similarly, therapists can report to the nurses any changes in the patient's condition that they observe during their intervention.

## 5. Shared Education

Continuing education is essential in the medical field. Nurses and therapists can benefit from joint workshops or educational sessions to better understand the latest techniques, tools and approaches in the different areas of neurological rehabilitation.

## 6. Care coordination

To avoid patient fatigue and optimise rest periods, it is essential to coordinate interventions. For example, avoid having a speech therapy session directly following an intensive physiotherapy session.

## 7. Exit planning and follow-up

When the patient is ready to leave the ward or hospital, close collaboration is needed to establish a plan for post-hospital care. This may include recommendations for home therapies, assistive devices or modifications to the home.

Ultimately, collaboration between nurses and therapists not only improves outcomes for neurology patients; it also creates a more harmonious and productive working environment for all the professionals involved. Each specialist plays a distinct note, but together they create a symphony of care that can greatly improve a patient's quality of life.

# Case studies
# of successes in rehabilitation

Case studies are an effective way of showing in concrete terms how theory and practice come together to create positive outcomes for rehabilitation patients. Let's look at some fictional examples of success stories in neurological rehabilitation:

### 1. Mrs Dubois: Stroke rehabilitation
Initial situation :
Mrs Dubois, aged 68, was admitted to hospital following a stroke that paralysed the right side of her body. Initially, she was unable to walk, her speech was slurred, and she had difficulty performing simple tasks such as getting dressed.
Speech:
A multidisciplinary approach was adopted. Physiotherapy focused on muscle strengthening and mobility. Speech therapy addressed speech and swallowing problems. Occupational therapy helped to adapt his environment and teach him new methods for performing everyday tasks.
Issue :
After several months, Mrs Dubois was able to walk almost normally with the help of a cane, her speech improved considerably and she regained a degree of independence in her daily activities.

### 2. Mr Ahmed: Head injury following an accident
Initial situation :
Mr Ahmed, aged 32, suffered a serious head injury after a car accident. He had memory problems, mood swings and difficulty concentrating.
Speech:
A neuropsychologist worked with Mr Ahmed on his cognitive problems, while a rehabilitation therapist addressed motor deficits. Psychotherapy sessions were

also introduced to manage mood swings and post-traumatic stress.

Issue :

Over time, with constant support and targeted therapy, Mr Ahmed regained much of his cognitive ability, learned techniques for managing his stress and emotions, and gradually returned to work.

### 3. Miss Clara: Multiple sclerosis

Initial situation :

Miss Clara, 28, was diagnosed with multiple sclerosis (MS). She was experiencing numbness, coordination problems and extreme fatigue.

Speech:

Rehabilitation focused on managing fatigue, improving coordination and muscle strength. Interventions were also put in place to manage symptoms such as visual problems and heat sensitivity.

Issue :

Even though MS is a chronic disease, Clara has been able to maintain a satisfactory quality of life thanks to rehabilitation. She has adapted her lifestyle, incorporating periods of rest, but continues to work and participate in social activities, while successfully managing her symptoms.

These fictional case studies illustrate how rehabilitation, tailored to the specific needs of each patient, can greatly improve quality of life, restore lost function and help patients regain their independence, even after devastating medical events.

# Chapter 10:
# ETHICS AND DEONTOLOGY
# IN NEUROLOGY

## Ethical issues specific to neurology

Neurology, at the intersection of the brain, the mind and the body, is a field of major ethical dilemmas. Medical and technological advances regularly raise questions about respect for patients' dignity, rights and choices. Here are some of the ethical issues specific to neurology:

1. Definition of life and death:
   - **Vegetative state and minimally conscious state**: Determining whether a patient is conscious can influence crucial decisions such as continuing or stopping care. How can we be sure that a person is truly unconscious or without the potential to wake up?
   - **Definition of brain death**: The exact definition and criteria for declaring brain death vary from country to country, influencing decisions on organ donation or withdrawal of care.
2. Patient autonomy and decision-making:
   - **Informed consent**: In the context of neurological disorders, it can be difficult to determine whether a patient is capable of giving informed consent to a treatment or intervention.
   - **Patients suffering from dementia**: Changes in cognitive ability make therapeutic decision-making complex.

3. Innovative treatments and interventions:
   - **Deep brain stimulation**: Used to treat conditions such as Parkinson's disease, this procedure can change personality or behaviour. Who decides whether the benefits outweigh the potential risks?
   - **Neuroenhancement**: The use of drugs or interventions to improve or increase brain function in healthy individuals raises questions about fairness, social pressure and the limits of 'normality'.
4. Confidentiality and disclosure of information:
   - Genetic testing to identify the risk of neurodegenerative diseases (such as Huntington's disease) raises the question of whether, when and how to disclose this information to patients and their families.
5. Allocation of resources:
   - With limited resources, how do you decide on the distribution of expensive treatments or access to specialist interventions?
6. Clinical research:
   - The conduct of clinical trials in neurological patients, particularly those who cannot give consent, raises questions about the potential use and benefit-risk of interventions.
7. Relations with industry:
   - Collaborations between neurologists and the pharmaceutical or technology industries can create conflicts of interest, potentially influencing therapeutic choices or research directions.

As a discipline that studies the most complex organ in the human body, neurology is naturally faced with profound ethical dilemmas. Addressing these issues requires multidisciplinary thinking, involving not only neurologists, but also patients, families, ethicists and society as a whole.

# Patient rights and autonomy

Patients' rights in neurology, as in any other medical field, are fundamental to guaranteeing the dignity, respect and appropriate care of each individual. Autonomy, in particular, is a central pillar of these rights, ensuring that patients are in control of their own medical decisions. Let's explore these concepts in more detail.

Patients' rights

**1. Right to information**: All patients have the right to be informed in a clear manner, adapted to their level of understanding, about their state of health, the proposed interventions, their benefits and their potential risks.

**2. Right to informed consent**: No medical procedure or research may be carried out without the free and informed consent of the patient.

**3. Right to confidentiality**: All information concerning the patient, including his/her state of health, treatment and medical history, must remain confidential.

**4. Right of access to medical records**: Patients have the right to consult and obtain a copy of their medical records.

**5. Right to quality care**: Every patient has the right to receive the best possible care, adapted to their state of health and without discrimination.

**6. Right to refuse treatment**: Even after being informed of the possible consequences, a patient has the right to refuse treatment or an intervention.

**7. Right to complain** : If a patient feels that their rights have not been respected, they have the right to lodge a complaint.

Patient autonomy

Autonomy refers to the ability to make decisions and act according to one's own values and beliefs. In the medical context, this means respecting the patient's choices and decisions, even if they differ from what the healthcare professional believes to be 'best' for the patient.

- **Respect for patient choice**: Autonomy implies that patients have the final say on medical decisions affecting them, as long as they are able to understand the implications of these decisions.
- **Decision-making capacity**: In certain cases, such as severe neurological disorders, the patient's ability to make decisions may be compromised. In these situations, it may be necessary to appoint a legal representative or trusted person to make decisions on the patient's behalf.
- **Advance care planning**: Advance directives or living wills allow patients to express their wishes regarding the care and treatment they would like to receive (or not receive) if one day they are no longer able to communicate or make decisions.
- **Education and support**: To ensure independence, it is essential to educate patients about their condition and treatment options. Helping them understand their disease empowers them to make informed decisions.

Patients' rights and autonomy are essential to ensuring respectful, patient-centred medical care. In the field of neurology, with conditions that can affect decision-making capacity and cognition, these principles take on particular importance, requiring constant attention and sensitivity on the part of healthcare professionals.

# Case studies and common ethical dilemmas

Neurology, because of its close relationship with the brain and consciousness, is faced with a series of complex ethical dilemmas. Case studies offer an opportunity to examine these dilemmas in depth, enabling healthcare professionals to better navigate these delicate situations. Here are some examples of case studies, followed by the associated common ethical dilemmas.

Case studies:
1. Mrs Dupont, 78, advanced Alzheimer's disease:
Mrs Dupont, who lives in a long-term care facility, no longer recognises her family. She drew up advance directives ten years ago, refusing any invasive treatment. Now she has an infection that requires hospitalisation and possibly surgery. Should her instructions be followed, even if her family insists on treatment?
**Ethical dilemma**: Advance directives vs. the family's current wishes.

2. Mr Bernard, 40, head injury following an accident:
After a serious car accident, Mr Bernard is in a coma. Tests showed minimal brain activity. His wife, hoping for a miracle, insisted that he remain on mechanical ventilation. The medical team, however, believes that there is little chance of recovery.
**Ethical dilemma**: When to withdraw life support? Who decides?

3. Clara, 16, epilepsy:
Clara, recently diagnosed with epilepsy, wants to take part in all school and extra-curricular activities like her peers, including swimming. Her neurologist is concerned about the potential risks of having a seizure while swimming.
**Ethical dilemma**: patient autonomy vs. safety and well-being.

**Common ethical dilemmas:**
1. Stopping treatment:
In what circumstances is it appropriate to stop treatment, especially if this could lead to the patient's death? How can quality of life be balanced with longevity?

## 2. Informed consent:

How can informed consent be obtained for patients with cognitive difficulties or altered consciousness?

## 3. Clinical research:

When working with patients with neurological disorders, how do you ensure that they are genuinely able to give their consent to take part in a clinical study?

## 4. Neuroenhancement:

How ethical is it to use neurological interventions to 'improve' healthy individuals, rather than to treat disease?

## 5. Genetics and predictions:

Is it ethical to reveal to a patient that they have a genetic predisposition to a neurodegenerative disease with no known treatment?

In examining these cases and dilemmas, it is clear that neurology, like many medical specialties, is confronted with profound ethical issues. A multidisciplinary approach, which includes consultation with ethicists, patients, families and healthcare professionals, is often required to navigate these complex waters.

# Chapter 11:
# INNOVATIONS AND ADVANCES IN NEUROLOGY

## The latest discoveries and research

The field of neurology is constantly evolving, with new discoveries and research published almost daily. It's important to note that my last update was in September 2021. That said, here is an overview of the major advances up to that date:

1. Neurodegenerative diseases :
   - **Alzheimer's disease**: Progress has been made in identifying early biomarkers of the disease, facilitating early diagnosis. Aducanumab, a drug that targets amyloid plaques, has been approved by the FDA, although it remains controversial due to its uncertain clinical benefits.
   - **Parkinson's disease**: Research has focused on understanding the role of alpha-synuclein proteins and new targets for gene therapy.

2. Neuroinflammation :
Studies have highlighted the potential role of inflammation in various neurological diseases, including depression. Treatments targeting inflammatory pathways are currently under investigation.

3. Neuroplasticity :
Understanding the brain's ability to remodel itself and create new connections, even in adulthood, has opened up new avenues for innovative therapies, particularly for stroke victims.

4. Epilepsy :
Advances in implantable devices have offered new solutions for patients suffering from refractory epilepsy.

5. Gene therapies :
Gene therapies have been developed to treat certain rare neurological diseases, such as spinal muscular atrophy.

6. Brain-computer interfaces :
These technologies, which enable direct communication between the brain and external devices, have progressed, offering hope for patients who are paralysed or suffering from degenerative diseases.

7. Microbiome and the brain :
Research has revealed links between the gut microbiome and the brain, opening up potential new therapies for diseases such as multiple sclerosis and Parkinson's disease.

8. Head injuries :
The importance of the long-term consequences of head injuries, particularly in terms of the risk of dementia or neurodegenerative diseases, has become increasingly clear.

9. Neuroimaging :
Advanced imaging techniques, such as high-resolution functional MRI, have made it possible to visualise the brain in action with unprecedented precision.

10. Stem cell therapies :
Clinical trials have evaluated the potential of stem cells in the regeneration of damaged tissue, particularly in spinal cord injuries.

Advances in neurology are happening at a rapid pace. To stay up to date, it is crucial for professionals to regularly follow publications in major scientific journals, attend conferences and collaborate with experts in the field.

## The impact of innovative technologies (e.g. telemedicine, artificial intelligence)

The impact of innovative technologies in neurology is considerable, transforming the way care is delivered and diseases are diagnosed and treated. The applications of telemedicine and artificial intelligence (AI) are striking examples. Let's find out together how these technologies are influencing the neurological landscape.

Telemedicine :
The rapid adoption of telemedicine has been accelerated by global events, notably the COVID-19 pandemic. In neurology, this has been particularly beneficial for :
- **Remote consultations**: Patients with neurological diseases, particularly those living in remote areas, can access specialists without having to travel.
- **Telestroke**: The ability to quickly assess a patient suspected of having a stroke and collaborate with specialist centres can make all the difference in terms of patient outcomes.
- **Patient monitoring**: Telemedicine enables patients suffering from chronic illnesses such as Parkinson's disease or epilepsy to be monitored regularly, without having to travel frequently.

Artificial Intelligence (AI) :
AI, with its machine learning capabilities, is bringing about a revolution in neurology diagnosis, treatment and research.
- **Neuroimaging**: AI algorithms can detect subtle anomalies in brain images, sometimes long before

80

they are visible to the human eye. This can be crucial for the early diagnosis of diseases such as Alzheimer's.

- **Prediction and personalisation**: AI can help predict which patient will respond best to which treatment, enabling more personalised medicine.
- **Seizure detection**: For epilepsy patients, AI-based devices can continuously monitor and predict an impending seizure, offering a chance to take preventative action.
- **Brain-computer interfaces**: These devices, combined with AI, can help restore function in people with paralysis or other neurological deficits.
- **Research and clinical trials**: AI can rapidly analyse large datasets to find patterns or correlations, speeding up research and the discovery of new treatments.


Ethical and practical implications :
Although technology offers many opportunities, it also poses challenges. Data confidentiality, security and the ethical implications of automated decision-making are all issues that need to be carefully addressed.

Ongoing training for neurologists and healthcare professionals is also essential if they are to adapt to this new technological era. They must not only understand how to use these tools effectively, but also be aware of their limitations.
In short, the convergence of neurology with telemedicine and AI promises rapid advances in terms of patient care and research. However, this transition must be carefully managed to ensure the safety, ethics and effectiveness of the new methods.

# The neurology of tomorrow : prospects and challenges

Neurology, like many other medical fields, is at a crossroads. With rapid technological advances, advances in our understanding of the underlying mechanisms of neurological disease and the globalisation of healthcare, the prospects are exciting, but they also come with new challenges. Let's delve into the future of neurology to find out what lies ahead.

1. Personalised medicine:
Advances in genomic sequencing and data analysis promise more personalised treatments. Depending on their genetics, lifestyle and other factors, treatments could be tailored to the individual to maximise efficacy and minimise side effects.

2. Regenerative therapies:
Stem cells and gene therapies offer the hope of restoring function in neurodegenerative diseases and after traumatic injury to the nervous system.

3. Augmented reality and virtual reality:
These technologies could transform neurological rehabilitation, offering immersive simulations to help restore motor or cognitive function after stroke, head injury or other conditions.

4. Implantable devices:
In addition to the deep brain stimulators used in Parkinson's disease, we could see devices that improve memory, aid vision or restore other neurological functions.

5. Neuroethics:
With all these advances comes a new set of ethical questions. Who has access to these treatments? How

should sensitive patient data be handled? And to what extent should we interfere with the natural functioning of the human brain?

6. Health economics:
As treatments become more sophisticated, they also become more expensive. How will healthcare systems, insurance companies and patients themselves manage these costs?

7. Interdisciplinary collaboration:
Neurology can no longer function in a bubble. Collaboration with other medical disciplines, as well as with fields such as computer science, robotics and even the social sciences, will be crucial.

8. Education and training:
Neurologists and other healthcare professionals will need to constantly update their skills and knowledge, not only in neurology, but also in technology, ethics and communication.

9. Overall access to care:
Disparity in access to neurological care, particularly in low- and middle-income countries, is a major concern. How can we ensure that the benefits of advances in neurology reach everyone, regardless of geography or wealth?

10. Environment and neurology:
With climate change and environmental concerns, emerging diseases and challenges to neurological health could arise.

The neurology of tomorrow offers incredible opportunities to improve patients' lives. However, each advance brings its own set of challenges. Meeting them will require enlightened vision, unprecedented collaboration and a commitment to ethics and fairness. Neurology is on the cusp of a revolution, and we must be prepared to navigate its often uncharted waters.

# Chapter 12:
## THE IMPORTANCE OF INTERDISCIPLINARY WORK

## Collaborate
## with other medical specialities

Although neurology focuses on the diagnosis and treatment of diseases of the nervous system, it does not operate in a vacuum. In fact, caring for neurology patients often requires close collaboration with other medical specialities in order to provide comprehensive, holistic care. Let's look at how this collaboration manifests itself in the day-to-day work of a neurologist and why it is crucial to optimal care.

Cardiology:
Cardiovascular disorders have direct implications for neurological health. For example, a patient who has suffered a stroke needs to work with a cardiologist to manage the risk factors, such as arrhythmia or hypertension, that may have contributed to the stroke.

Psychiatry:
Neurological diseases can often have psychiatric manifestations. For example, depression is common in patients with Parkinson's disease. Collaboration with psychiatry can help to diagnose and treat these symptoms.

Neurosurgery:
Some conditions, such as brain tumours or aneurysms, may require surgery. Neurologists often work hand in hand with neurosurgeons to discuss the best options for the patient.

Radiology:
Neuroimaging is fundamental to the diagnosis of many neurological diseases. Neurologists work with radiologists to interpret MRI, CT, PET and other images.

Rheumatology:
Autoimmune diseases, such as multiple sclerosis, often overlap with rheumatology and neurology. Joint management can benefit patients.

Endocrinology:
Hormonal imbalances can influence or mimic neurological diseases. Thyroid disorders, for example, can cause neuropathy or myopathy.

Medical genetics:
Many neurological diseases have a genetic component. Working with medical geneticists can help identify risks, advise patients and guide treatment.

Re-education and rehabilitation:
After events such as a stroke or traumatic brain injury, patients may require physiotherapy, occupational therapy or speech therapy to regain function. Neurologists work closely with these professionals to ensure optimal recovery.
Gerontology:

As people age, neurodegenerative diseases such as Alzheimer's become more common. Collaboration with gerontologists can help to manage the specific challenges faced by elderly patients.

Interdisciplinary collaboration enables comprehensive care to be provided, with each specialist contributing his or her unique expertise to offer the best possible care to the patient. This requires open communication, respect for each other's contributions and a constant desire to put the patient at the centre of everything we do. In today's complex medical landscape, teamwork is more crucial than ever.

# Complementary roles within the team

Caring for a patient, particularly in a field as complex as neurology, is far from being the effort of a single individual. Instead, it requires fluid and complementary coordination between different healthcare professionals. Each member of the team plays a distinct role, and it is the synergy of their skills that ensures comprehensive patient care. Let's explore how these roles complement each other in a neurology team.

1. Neurologists:
They are often the "conductors" who diagnose neurological diseases, propose treatment plans and supervise the patient's overall care.

2. Nurses specialising in neurology:
They are often the first responders to any changes in the patient's condition. They administer medication, monitor vital signs, educate patients and their families and act as a bridge between the patient and the neurologist.

3. Neurosurgeons:
They intervene when surgical treatment is necessary, whether to remove a tumour, treat an aneurysm or implant a device.

4. Radiologists:
Essential for imaging the brain and spine, they provide detailed interpretations of images to guide diagnosis and treatment.

5. Physiotherapists:
They work with patients to improve mobility, strengthen muscles and restore functions lost as a result of neurological conditions.

6. Speech therapists:
Crucial for patients with speech or swallowing problems, often following a stroke.

7. Occupational therapists:
They help patients regain their independence in everyday activities, such as dressing, cooking and working.

8. Psychologists and psychiatrists:
They address the emotional and mental aspects of neurological illness, offering support, coping strategies and, if necessary, treatment.

9. Social workers:
They help navigate non-medical challenges, such as discharge planning, home accessibility and financial issues.

10. Pharmacists:
They advise on the administration of medicines, possible interactions and side effects.

11. Nutritionists:
Some neurological disorders may require dietary adjustments or specific diets. Nutritionists guide these changes to ensure optimal health.

The beauty lies in the way these roles intersect and complement each other. For example, when a patient is recovering from a stroke, they may need a neurologist to manage their medical treatment, a physiotherapist to restore mobility, a speech therapist to help them speak again, and a social worker to organise care at home.

This complementary approach ensures that every aspect of the patient's well-being is taken into account. It reflects a holistic view of health, where the patient is seen as a whole, and not just through the prism of their illness. It is a truly patient-centred approach, where the aim is not just to treat an illness, but to restore quality of life.

# The benefits a holistic approach to care

The holistic approach to medical care was born of the realisation that human beings are not simply aggregates of symptoms and diseases, but complex, interconnected entities that require attention to all their facets if they are to be truly healed. Far from being just a philosophical concept, this approach brings tangible benefits to patient care, particularly in areas as sensitive as neurology. Let's take a look at these benefits together.

1. Individualised care:
Each individual is unique, with his or her own background, environment and life experiences. The holistic approach recognises this uniqueness and adjusts care accordingly, ensuring that each patient receives the treatment best suited to their situation.

2. Emotional and mental well-being:
Focusing solely on the physical medical problem can miss the emotional and mental distress. A holistic approach ensures that these aspects are also addressed, which can have a profound impact on healing and quality of life.

3. Promoting prevention:
Rather than focusing solely on treating existing illnesses, the holistic approach also emphasises the importance of prevention, addressing elements such as lifestyle, nutrition and stress management.

4. Integration of complementary medicine:
Many patients find relief or support in complementary therapies such as acupuncture, meditation or herbal medicine. The holistic approach recognises and integrates these therapies where deemed beneficial.

5. Improving the patient/carer relationship:
By seeking to understand the whole patient, a deeper and more meaningful relationship is often established between patient and carer. This can improve communication, build trust and ultimately improve care outcomes.

6. Managing complex symptoms:
Some symptoms cannot be easily explained by a single physical cause. A holistic view can help to identify and treat underlying or interconnected causes that might be overlooked in a more reductionist approach.

7. Reinforcing patient autonomy:
The holistic approach often encourages patients to take an active part in their own healing, by educating them and involving them in therapeutic decisions.

8. Reduction in readmissions and complications:
By addressing the root causes and integrating various treatment modalities, the holistic approach can reduce the chances of recurrence or subsequent complications.

9. Increased patient satisfaction:
Patients who feel listened to, understood and cared for in every dimension of their being tend to be more satisfied with their care.

Ultimately, the holistic approach reflects a broad vision of health, recognising that our well-being is the product of a multitude of interdependent factors. By integrating this vision into medical practice, we can hope not only to treat disease, but also to promote true and lasting health.

# Chapter 13:
# HEALTH AND WELL-BEING
# OF THE NEUROLOGY NURSE

## Recognise and prevent burnout

Burnout is a syndrome resulting from chronic stress at work that has not been adequately managed. It is particularly prevalent in the healthcare professions, where workers are often faced with emotionally charged situations, long and irregular working hours, and constant pressure to provide high-quality care. Recognising the early signs and putting preventive measures in place is crucial to ensuring the well-being of carers and the quality of patient care.

Recognising the signs of burnout:
- **Emotional exhaustion**: Feeling drained, exhausted by work, with no energy or enthusiasm to start a new day.
- **Depersonalisation**: The development of a feeling of distance or cynicism towards work, colleagues or patients.
- **Decreased sense of personal accomplishment**: Feeling that what you do is unimportant or of no value, or perception of diminished professional skills.
- **Physical symptoms**: Trouble sleeping, headaches, digestive problems, muscle pain, and increased susceptibility to illness.
- **Mood changes**: Irritability, sadness, apathy or even depressive symptoms.
- **Withdrawal**: Decreased social or professional involvement, avoidance of responsibilities, or increased absence from work.

Preventive measures against burnout:

- **Work-life balance**: Encourage and respect a balance between work and personal time, allowing for recuperation and relaxation.
- **Social support**: Creating a working environment where colleagues support each other, share experiences and find comfort in camaraderie.
- **Supervision and mentoring**: For new employees or those facing new challenges, having a mentor or regular supervision can help navigate professional challenges.
- **Stress management training**: This can include relaxation techniques, meditation, or even practices such as yoga or tai chi.
- **Recognition and appreciation**: Feeling valued and appreciated in your role can make a huge difference to how you perceive your work.
- **Opportunity for feedback**: Provide channels for employees to express their concerns, suggestions or frustrations.
- **Limiting overtime**: Ensuring that staff are not constantly overworked, and ensuring that there is sufficient recovery time between shifts.
- **Mental health resources**: Provide access to counselling services or mental health support programmes for staff.
- **Ongoing training**: Invest in ongoing training for staff to ensure they feel competent and up to date in their skills.
- **Taking breaks**: Regular breaks during the day to relax, get some fresh air or simply switch off for a few minutes can be revitalising.

Recognising and preventing burnout is essential not only for the well-being of healthcare professionals, but also to ensure that patients receive optimum care. An exhausted carer is less effective, more likely to make mistakes and can potentially affect the quality of care provided. By investing in the well-being of carers, we are also investing in the health and well-being of the patients they serve.

# Stress management strategies

Stress management is a key element in ensuring the mental and physical well-being of carers, particularly in the demanding field of neurology. Uncontrolled stress can lead to reduced performance, increased susceptibility to errors and, in the long term, chronic health problems. Implementing effective stress management strategies is therefore crucial to the health of carers and the quality of patient care.

Cognitive and behavioural methods:
- **Recognising your own stress signals**: Take the time to assess yourself regularly to recognise the first signs of stress. This allows you to take action before the stress becomes overwhelming.
- **Reviewing expectations**: Strive to set realistic expectations for yourself and others, avoid perfection at all costs.
- **Time management**: Organise and prioritise tasks to avoid feeling overwhelmed. Make lists, set priorities and delegate where possible.
- **Reflecting on and challenging negative thoughts**: When you find yourself thinking negatively, it's important to challenge these thoughts and replace them with positive affirmations.

Relaxation techniques:
- **Deep breathing**: The simple act of taking several deep breaths can help reduce feelings of anxiety.

- **Meditation and mindfulness**: These techniques help you focus on the present moment, reduce intrusive thoughts and relax.
- **Visualisation techniques**: Imagining a soothing place or situation can help you to relax mentally.
- **Stretching exercises**: Even a few simple stretches can help relieve muscle tension.

Lifestyle habits:
- **Regular exercise**: Physical activity releases endorphins, brain chemicals that act like natural painkillers.
- **Balanced diet**: A healthy diet can help regulate mood and build resilience in the face of stress.
- **Adequate sleep** : Sleep is essential for physical and mental recovery.
- **Limit caffeine and sugar**: These stimulants can increase anxiety.

Social and emotional support:
- **Talk to someone you trust**: Discussing your concerns with a colleague, friend, family member or professional can help put things into perspective.
- **Participating in support groups**: Sometimes sharing your experiences with others in the same situation can be beneficial.
- **Leisure**: Finding time for activities you enjoy can be a breath of fresh air.
- **Holidays**: Even a short break from work can help you recharge your batteries.
- **Sessions with a therapist or counsellor**: For some people, talking to a professional can provide additional tools and strategies for managing stress.

Stress is a natural response to the challenges and pressures of everyday life, but managing it effectively is essential for health and well-being. Everyone is different, and what works for one person may not work for another. So it's important to experiment with different strategies to find the ones that work best for you.

# The balance professional-personal life

Work-life balance is a major concern for many professionals, particularly in demanding fields such as neurology. It's not just a question of individual well-being, although that's crucial, but also a question of the quality of care provided to patients. An exhausted, overworked or emotionally drained carer cannot provide the best possible care.

Why is balance so crucial?
In neurology, as in many other areas of medicine, the days can be long, the cases complex and the emotions high. There's the pain of seeing a patient suffer, the stress of unexpected emergencies, the pressure to keep up to date with the latest research and techniques, and many other factors that can make this profession particularly challenging.

What's more, outside the hospital or clinic, life goes on. Nurses have families, friends, passions and hobbies that also demand their attention and energy. Ignoring one aspect of life in favour of another can lead to a loss of meaning, resentment, exhaustion or even mental health problems.

Striking a balance:
- **Prioritise:** It is essential to determine what is really important in your life and to devote time to these priorities. This could mean refusing overtime, delegating certain tasks or asking for help when necessary.

- **Setting limits**: It's crucial to be clear about what you are and aren't prepared to accept at work. This could mean not answering work emails at home or taking regular breaks during the working day.
- **Taking care of yourself**: Self-care is not a luxury, but a necessity. This could mean exercising, meditating, reading, or any other activity that recharges the batteries.
- **Asking for help**: Sometimes, despite your best efforts, it can be difficult to maintain balance. At such times, it's essential to seek support, whether from colleagues, mentors, therapists or coaches.
- **Be flexible**: Life changes, and so do an individual's needs and priorities. It's crucial to regularly review and adjust your work-life balance to reflect these changes.

Striking a balance between professional and personal life is not always easy, especially in a field as demanding as neurology. However, with thought, support and constant attention to one's needs and priorities, it is possible to find a balance that works for you and your patients.

# Chapter 14:
# CAREER DEVELOPMENT AND SKILLS DEVELOPMENT

## Continuing education in neurology

Continuing education in neurology
In its never-ending quest to understand and improve, medicine is constantly evolving. In neurology, where one of the most complex systems in the human body is being explored, this evolution is all the more rapid and profound. In this context, continuing education is not only recommended but essential for all professionals, and in particular for nurses specialising in neurology.

The need to update
Neurology, like many other medical disciplines, is characterised by an abundance of research and discoveries. Whether it's new imaging techniques, advances in the treatment of neurodegenerative diseases or unravelling the mysteries of cognition, the field is constantly expanding. For nurses, staying up to date means being able to offer the best possible care, using the most advanced techniques and the most effective treatments.

Continuing training arrangements
- **Seminars and conferences**: These meetings are not just about learning, but also about discussing and exchanging experiences with peers and experts in the field.
- **Specialist     publications**: Neurology journals and newspapers are invaluable sources of information on the latest research and discoveries.

- **Practical workshops**: These sessions enable nurses to familiarise themselves with new techniques or equipment.
- **E-learning**: With the advent of digital technologies, a large number of online training modules are now available, allowing flexible learning.
- **Specialist certifications**: Obtaining certification in a neurology subspecialty can not only deepen knowledge, but also enhance a nurse's professionalism.

The importance of professional curiosity
Beyond technical knowledge, continuing education cultivates professional curiosity, which is essential in a field as complex as neurology. This curiosity encourages nurses to ask questions, look for solutions, challenge themselves, and ultimately offer better quality care.

Continuing education in neurology is a proactive approach to staying at the cutting edge of the discipline. It ensures that nurses do not rest on their laurels, but constantly seek to improve their practice, for the benefit of their patients and the advancement of their careers. Ultimately, in the dynamic and ever-changing world of neurology, learning is truly a never-ending journey.

# Integration of new technologies

Integration of new technologies in neurology
Neurology, like many other branches of medicine, is constantly evolving thanks to the advent of new technologies. These innovations, ranging from AI to cutting-edge medical devices, have significantly transformed patient care, diagnosis and treatment of neurological conditions. The integration of these technologies is not without its challenges, but it paves the

way for more precise, more effective and sometimes less invasive care.

The advent of advanced imaging
Neurology has always depended on imaging techniques to visualise the brain and nervous system. Today, thanks to technological advances, techniques such as functional MRI, positron emission tomography (PET) and magnetoencephalography offer detailed views of brain activity, enabling a deeper understanding of pathologies.

The age of artificial intelligence (AI)
AI and machine learning have found their place in neurology, particularly in the interpretation of brain scans, the prediction of disease progression and the personalisation of treatments. Algorithms can now detect subtle anomalies in brain images, sometimes even before symptoms appear.

Telemedicine and remote care
The COVID-19 pandemic has increased the use of telemedicine. For patients suffering from neurological diseases, this has meant regular consultations without the stress and fatigue of travelling, especially for those with reduced mobility.

Connected medical devices
Devices such as portable electroencephalograms, wearables that track neurological parameters, and programmable drug pumps offer real-time monitoring of patients, enabling treatments to be tailored to specific needs.

Robot-assisted surgery
In delicate procedures such as brain surgery, AI-assisted robots provide unrivalled precision, minimising risks and improving post-operative outcomes.

Challenges and ethical considerations
While these technologies offer new opportunities, they also come with their share of challenges. Issues of data confidentiality, equity of access to care and adequate training of healthcare professionals are at the heart of these concerns. In addition, over-reliance on technology can risk overshadowing the importance of clinical examination and human interaction.

The integration of new technologies in neurology is an exciting journey, offering incredible opportunities to improve patient care. For nurses, this means constant training, adaptation and curiosity. But with these tools at our fingertips, the potential for delivering superior care has never been greater.

# The importance of research in neurology for nurses

The importance of neurological research for nurses
Research in neurology is a constantly evolving dynamic, seeking to demystify the complexities of the nervous system, elucidate the mechanisms of neurological diseases and develop new treatments and interventions. For neurology nurses, research is much more than just scientific news: it is an essential pillar of clinical practice and a key factor in improving patient care.

Informing clinical practice
Research discoveries provide scientific evidence to guide nursing care. They offer evidence-based answers about the best interventions, new therapies and even the best ways to communicate with patients. By engaging in research, nurses can refine their practice to provide more effective, patient-centred care.

Anticipating and adapting to change
The field of neurology is evolving rapidly. Nurses who are up to date with current research are better prepared to anticipate their patients' future needs, adapt to new protocols and integrate new technologies or treatment methods.

Improving the quality of care
Research provides crucial information on patient outcomes, enabling best practice to be identified, areas for improvement to be recognised and changes to be initiated to improve the quality and safety of care.
Contributing to the profession

Nurses are not just consumers of research, but can also play a key role in carrying it out. By participating in studies, collecting data or even initiating research projects, nurses contribute to the advancement of the profession, thereby enriching nursing knowledge in neurology.

Advocating for patients
A thorough understanding of research enables nurses to advocate on behalf of patients' needs and interests. They can advise on the most appropriate treatments, educate patients about the options available, and even influence policies and practices within medical institutions.

Research in neurology is invaluable for nurses. It strengthens their practice, equips them for optimal care and positions them as a major player in improving neurological care. By embracing research and actively engaging in this quest for knowledge, neurology nurses are not just keeping up with progress; they are shaping it.

# Chapter 15:
# TESTIMONIALS AND CASE STUDIES

## Case studies
## Experiences of neurology nurses

### 1. An unexpected connection :

Sarah, a young neurology nurse, was assigned to Mr Dupont, a 60-year-old man recently diagnosed with Parkinson's disease. Despite the tremors and rigidity, what affected Sarah most was Mr Dupont's emotional isolation. One day, she brought in an old guitar and encouraged Mr Dupont to play, remembering that he had told her about his love of music. The musical sessions became a routine, not only helping Mr Dupont to improve his fine motor skills, but also reconnecting him with a forgotten passion, thereby reducing his depressive symptoms.

### 2. The importance of listening :

Marc, an experienced nurse, was looking after Mrs Lefevre, who had advanced multiple sclerosis. One morning, when she seemed particularly distracted, Marc sat down beside her, holding her hand. After a long silence, Mrs Lefevre confided her fear of becoming a burden on her family. By taking the time to listen and reassure, Marc was able to organise family therapy sessions to address these concerns, thereby strengthening the family bond.

### 3. A sure sign :

Élise had always been good at observing the little details in her patients. One day, while making a tour of the rooms, she noticed a slight droop in the face of Mr Bernard, an otherwise healthy patient. Recognising this as a potential sign of stroke, she immediately alerted the medical team.

Her quick actions led to immediate intervention, minimising brain damage and giving Mr Bernard a better chance of recovery.

**4. Discovering a vocation :**
Julien, initially a cardiology nurse, was temporarily transferred to neurology due to staff shortages. During his time there, he was deeply affected by the complexity of care and the intellectual challenge of understanding the nervous system. One epilepsy patient in particular inspired him with his resilience. Faced with an unexpected seizure, Julien followed procedures, reassuring the patient throughout. This experience led him to specialise in neurology, recognising the depth and richness of this speciality.

Every day, neurology nurses face challenges that require not only clinical expertise, but also deep compassion, active listening and adaptability. These case studies show the depth of their impact, making a difference to patients' lives through simple gestures, careful observation or decisive action.

# Lessons from complex situations

The neurology ward, with its mysteries and challenges, offers many situations that test the skills, resilience and empathy of carers. These situations, though difficult, also offer invaluable lessons for nurses. Here are a few lessons from these complex moments.

1. Every patient is unique:
When Caroline started working in neurology, she quickly learned that two patients with the same disease can react very differently. One patient with Parkinson's may be optimistic and combative, while another may sink into

depression. The lesson? It is essential to approach each patient as an individual and to personalise care.

2. Patience is essential:
Alexandre, a nurse, found it difficult to communicate with a patient suffering from aphasia following a stroke. After several frustrating attempts to understand the patient's needs, Alexandre realised that he needed to slow down, be patient and use non-verbal methods to establish a connection. This experience taught him the importance of patience in neurology, where communication deficits are common.

3. The importance of teamwork :
Sophie found herself overwhelmed by a patient with multiple sclerosis whose symptoms were worsening rapidly. She quickly realised that she couldn't manage everything on her own. By working closely with neurologists, physiotherapists and social workers, Sophie was able to create an integrative care plan for the patient. The lesson? Interdisciplinary collaboration is essential to meet the complex needs of neurological patients.

4. Flexibility is a strength:
When Éric was faced with an epilepsy patient whose seizures were not responding to the usual medication, he had to quickly adapt his approach. Working with the medical team, they explored other treatment options and adjusted the medication regime. This reinforced Éric's belief that flexibility and adaptability are crucial in neurology.

5. Dignity comes first :
Nadine remembers a patient with Alzheimer's who found it difficult to carry out simple tasks. Instead of doing these tasks for herself, Nadine took the time to patiently guide the patient, preserving her dignity and independence. She

learned that even in the most difficult of times, it is essential to treat every patient with respect and dignity.

Neurology is a field where uncertainties abound, and nurses are often faced with situations where there are no clear answers. However, these challenges also offer the opportunity to learn and grow as a healthcare professional, strengthening the ability to provide exceptional care, even in the most complex situations.

# Anecdotes and inspiring moments

The world of neurology is not only full of mysteries and challenges, it's also full of touching and inspiring moments. These anecdotes, often from the heart of the neurology department, remind us why so many nurses are passionate about this field.

1. Jeanne's dance :
Jeanne, aged 70, had been suffering from Parkinson's disease for several years. Despite her rigidity and tremors, she often spoke nostalgically of her passion for dancing. One day, one of her nurses, Léa, put on a song from her era and offered her her hand. Together, they danced in the hospital corridor. Jeanne, her eyes shining, showed that illness cannot always steal joy.

2. Samuel's smile :
Samuel, a young man of 25, was recovering from a serious car accident. He had become a quadriplegic. Every day, Sarah, his nurse, encouraged him with exercises and conversation. One morning, Samuel moved his toe. This small movement, symbolising hope and the potential for recovery, was celebrated with tears and laughter by the whole ward.

3. Lucie's notebook :

Lucie, who had a brain tumour, knew that she would gradually lose her memory. Rather than give in to sadness, she decided, with the help of her nurse Claire, to create a notebook. Every day, they wrote down memories, stories and photos. The notebook became a treasure for Lucie and her family, preserving precious moments despite her illness.

4. The return of the voice :

Following a stroke, Marc had lost the ability to speak. He communicated in frustration through gestures and looks. His nurse, Fatima, worked tirelessly with him, using speech therapy exercises and even playing recordings of his own voice. One day, Marc whispered a simple "thank you". That emotionally charged word was the start of his road to recovery.

5. Unexpected friendship :

Two patients, Pierre and Ahmed, one suffering from Alzheimer's disease and the other from multiple sclerosis, became friends in a shared room. Despite their cultural differences and the language barrier, they found comfort in each other. They laughed, played cards and supported each other. Their friendship reminded all the staff that compassion and understanding transcend all barriers.

Stories of triumphs large and small, moments of tenderness and human resilience punctuate the journey of every neurology nurse. These anecdotes remind us of the importance of empathy, perseverance and hope in the medical world, and reinforce the desire to provide care with heart and passion.

# Chapter 16:
# CONCLUSION
# AND FUTURE PROSPECTS

## The impact of technological progress and scientific approach to neurology

At the dawn of the 21st century, the field of neurology has witnessed a series of breathtaking breakthroughs, all made possible by technological and scientific progress. These advances have not only changed the way we understand the brain, but have also influenced approaches to treating and caring for patients.

1. Neuroimaging :
The emergence of advanced imaging techniques such as functional MRI (fMRI) and positron emission tomography (PET) has revolutionised our understanding of the brain in action. These tools have enabled doctors to 'see' brain activity in real time, identify specific areas of the brain responsible for different functions and detect abnormalities at very early stages of the disease.

2. Neuromodulation :
Devices such as deep brain stimulators, initially developed to treat Parkinson's disease, have shown potential in the treatment of other neurological conditions, such as obsessive-compulsive disorder or resistant depression. These interventions, which modify the brain's electrical activity, can improve patients' quality of life where drugs have failed.

3. Telemedicine :
With the exponential growth of digital technology, telemedicine has enabled neurologists to reach patients in remote areas, offering consultations, follow-ups and even certain forms of therapy at a distance. This is particularly valuable for patients with degenerative diseases who find it difficult to travel frequently.

4. Genetics and personalised medicine :
The ability to sequence DNA at an affordable cost has opened the way to more personalised treatments in neurology. Targeted gene therapies are being developed for diseases such as muscular dystrophy and certain forms of genetic blindness.

5. Brain Machine Interfaces (BMI) :
These devices, still in their infancy, promise to transform the lives of paralysed patients. They make it possible to transform brain activity into commands for external devices, enabling a quadriplegic patient, for example, to control an exoskeleton or a computer simply by thinking.

The intersection of technological progress and neurological science has led to an era of optimism and innovation. As well as improving diagnostic and therapeutic accuracy, these advances are increasing the hope of curing diseases once considered incurable. For nurses and all healthcare professionals, this means ongoing training, adaptation to new tools and methods, but above all, an unparalleled opportunity to improve patients' lives.

## Future vision of the nurse's role in neurology

The global medical landscape is undergoing unprecedented change, and the field of neurology is no exception. As technology advances and our knowledge of the brain expands, the role of the neurology nurse is also evolving. On the horizon, we can anticipate several trends that will influence this role.

1. Continuing education and training :
In the information age, learning never stops. Nurses will need to be at the forefront of new discoveries and technologies, requiring ongoing training and regular updates on the latest techniques, drugs and procedures.

2. Increased specialisation :
Like medicine itself, nursing is likely to see an increase in sub-specialisation. Nurses specialising in specific areas of neurology, such as movement disorders, degenerative diseases or paediatric conditions, could become commonplace.

3. Technological integration :
Nurses will be using more and more technologies in their care, from remote patient monitoring to the use of applications and devices to improve patients' quality of life. This integration will require both technical expertise and the ability to adapt to new tools.

4. Interdisciplinary collaboration :
The neurology nurse will increasingly be working with a diverse team: neurologists, therapists, social workers and even biomedical engineers. This interdisciplinary collaboration will be essential to ensure comprehensive patient care.

5. Expanded role in research :
Nurses will have the opportunity, and in some cases the responsibility, to participate actively in clinical research. Their direct and continuous interaction with patients makes them privileged observers of the effects of treatments and unmet care needs.

6. Holistic and preventive care :
With a better understanding of the social, environmental and genetic factors influencing neurological diseases, nurses will play a greater role in disease prevention and health promotion, adopting a holistic approach that takes into account the whole person.

Neurology, like all areas of medicine, is constantly evolving. Nurses, as a central pillar of the healthcare system, must adapt and evolve accordingly. Although the challenges are many, the future also promises vast opportunities for nurses to strengthen their impact, broaden their skills and play a key role in improving the quality of life of neurological patients.

# Encouraging the new generation

Neurology, one of the most fascinating and ever-evolving areas of medicine, promises great opportunities for the next generation of nurses. But, as with any demanding profession, it is essential to encourage, inspire and support aspiring neurology nurses to reach their full potential.

1. Encouraging passion and curiosity :
Every future neurology nurse carries within them a passion for understanding the complex workings of the nervous system. This passion, combined with an insatiable curiosity, is the cornerstone of success in this field. Let's encourage them to ask questions, pursue further training and never stop learning.

2. Highlighting successes :
The inspiring stories of nurses who have made a difference to the lives of their patients, who have been involved in groundbreaking discoveries or who have simply overcome personal challenges, can serve as role models for young

people. These stories show that, despite the obstacles, positive impact is within reach.

3. Providing solid mentoring :
The value of a mentor in a nurse's career path cannot be underestimated. Mentors can offer advice, share experiences and guide young nurses through the complexities of neurology.

4. Embracing technology :
Today's generation was born into a digital world. By integrating innovative technologies into training and practice, we can not only improve care, but also attract and retain the interest of young nurses.

5. Offer opportunities for professional development :
Workshops, seminars, scholarships and internships can provide aspiring nurses with the tools and skills they need to excel. Such opportunities can also give them an insight into the various possible specialisations in neurology.

6. Strengthening the sense of belonging :
Create an environment where everyone feels valued, supported and heard. Encourage mutual support, collaboration and the sharing of experiences within the nursing community.

The new generation of neurology nurses has the potential to push back the boundaries of what we know and what we can achieve in care. As healthcare professionals, educators and mentors, it is our duty to encourage, support and inspire these bright young minds. Tomorrow's neurology depends on the seeds we plant today.

# Glossary of medical terms

This glossary is not exhaustive and is for illustrative purposes only. For complete coverage, further research and collaboration with medical experts will be required.

**1. Aphasia: A** disorder affecting the ability to speak or understand language, often as a result of brain damage.

**2. Atrophy:** Reduction in the size or volume of a part of the body, here often used to describe a reduction in the size of the brain or its parts.

**3. Axon**: Extension of neurons used to conduct nerve impulses.

**4. Dementia**: Progressive decline in cognitive abilities, interfering with daily life.

**5. Dysarthria**: Difficulty in articulating words due to muscle weakness.

**6. EEG (Electroencephalogram)** : A test that measures the electrical activity of the brain.

**7. Encephalopathy**: General term for a disease that affects the function or structure of the brain.

**8. Hemiparesis**: Weakness or paralysis of one side of the body.

**9. MRI (Magnetic Resonance Imaging)** : Imaging technique used to visualise the inside of the body, particularly the brain.

**10. Meninges**: Membranes enveloping the brain and spinal cord.

**11. Neuron**: Nerve cell specialising in the transmission of information.

**12. Neurotransmitter**: chemical substance which transmits nerve impulses between neurons.

**13. Paresis**: Reduction in muscle mobility, ranging from weakness to paralysis.

**14. Synapse:** Junction zone between two neurons where nerve impulses are transmitted.

**15. CT (computed tomography):** imaging technique using X-rays to obtain detailed images of the body.

**16. Tremor**: Involuntary, rhythmic movement of a part of the body.

**17. Ventricles**: Cavities in the brain containing cerebrospinal fluid.

**18. Myelin:** Sheath surrounding certain axons, facilitating the transmission of nerve impulses.

**19. Plaque**: Abnormal accumulation of proteins in the brain, often associated with Alzheimer's disease.

**20. Sclerosis**: Hardening or scarring of tissues, as in multiple sclerosis, where the myelin of the central nervous system is attacked.

This glossary may be enriched by the addition of other important terms specific to neurology or neurology nursing practice. Collaboration with specialists in the field would be essential to ensure accuracy and completeness.

# Further reading and resources

Continuing education and self-instruction is essential for the neurology nurse, in order to keep up to date with the latest practices, discoveries and technologies. Here is a list of recommended resources and reading, which can be used as a starting point to enrich your knowledge:

Reference books :
- *Neurology for Nurses* by Jane Williams - A comprehensive exploration of neurological diseases, tailored to nursing practice.
- *The Basics of Neuroscience* by Mark F. Bear, Barry W. Connors, Michael A. Paradiso - An in-depth introduction to basic neuroscience.

Trade journals :
- *The Journal of Neuroscience Nursing* - Publishes articles on current research, evidence-based practice and specific cases in neuroscience nursing.
- *Neurology Clinical Practice - Features* articles on clinical practice in neurology, including nursing.

Websites :
- *World Federation of Neuroscience Nurses (WFNN)* - An organisation that supports neuroscience nurses worldwide.
- *American Association of Neuroscience Nurses (AANN)* - Provides resources, training and information on the latest research.

Webinars and online courses :
- *Neurology Nursing Certification Review* - A course designed to help nurses prepare for neurology certification.
- *Coursera & edX* - These platforms offer courses on a variety of subjects, including neurology and nursing.

Conferences and seminars :

*Annual Meeting of the European Association of Neuroscience Nurses (EANN)* - An opportunity to learn, network and discover the latest trends in neurology.

*International Conference on Alzheimer's & Parkinson's Diseases* - A major conference for those interested in degenerative diseases.

Others :

*Handbook of neurological protocols for nurses* - A practical guide to the day-to-day management of neurological patients.

Neurology *podcasts* - A modern way to learn on the move. There are several podcasts dedicated to neurology, its discoveries and clinical practice.

**Here is a list of resources and recommended reading for neurology nurses in the French-speaking world:**

Reference books :

*Précis de neurologie* by Paul Macé - A comprehensive exploration of neurological diseases, tailored for healthcare professionals.

*Fondements des neurosciences* by Bernard Bioulac and Michel Pêlegrini-Issac - A detailed introduction to neuroscience.

*Nursing practice in neurology* - A guide dedicated specifically to nursing practice in the neurological field.

Trade journals :

*Revue Neurologique* - A clinical and scientific journal dedicated to neuroscience.

*La Lettre du Neurologue* - Newsletter focusing on news and advances in the field of neurology.

Websites :

- *Société Française de Neurologie (SFN)* - Provides resources, news, training and information on the latest research in neurology.
- *Association des Neurologues Libéraux de Langue Française (ANLLF)* - Resources and news for neurologists and associated professionals.

Webinars and online training :

- *Université Numérique Francophone Mondiale* - This platform offers training modules dedicated to healthcare professionals, including neurology professionals.
- *Online nursing courses* - Many French-speaking institutions offer MOOCs and other distance learning courses for nurses.

Conferences and seminars :

- *Congress of the French Society of Neurology* - An annual event bringing together many professionals in the field.
- *Journées de Neurologie de Langue Française* - Lectures, workshops and presentations on the latest discoveries and practices in neurology.

Others :

- *Protocol manuals and practical guides* dedicated to neurology care - Some specialist health publishers regularly produce practical books for nurses.
- *Podcasts* on neurology in French - More and more platforms are offering audio content on medical topics so you can learn on the move.

Joining professional associations is also recommended, as they often offer resources, training and networking opportunities for professionals. Finally, the importance of on-the-job experience cannot be underestimated; working closely with mentors and experienced colleagues is an excellent way to learn and grow professionally.